What is Paranormal?

"A layman will no doubt find it hard to understand how pathological disorders of the body and mind can be eliminated by 'mere' words. He will feel that he is being asked to believe in magic. And he will not be so very wrong for the words which we use in our everyday speech are nothing more than watered down magic." (Freud)

This book provides further developments of such ideas, including Freud's uncanny, Jung's synchronicity, Daniels' transpersonal, Clarke's mindfulness and Sollod's anomalous experiences. The paranormal could be seen as being fundamental to the psychological therapies. Occasionally a writer brings this potential to our attention but questions of science, evidence-based practice etc. continue to dominate. Yet does this continue to lead to 'what's denied running even more wild'? Further, might the lessening of the paranormal be primarily what is lost, the aura, through the increase in internet therapy?

The question of the paranormal and the psychological therapies continues to persist, not only for psychoanalysis but the psychological therapies in general. This book attempts to address that.

The chapters in this book, apart from a new introduction and a new chapter, were originally published in the *European Journal of Psychotherapy and Counselling*.

Del Loewenthal is Emeritus Professor of Psychotherapy and Counselling at the University of Roehampton and is Chair of the Southern Association for Psychotherapy and Counselling (SAFPAC), London, UK. He is an existential-analytic psychotherapist and chartered psychologist, with a particular interest in phenomenology. His books include *Existential Psychotherapy and Counselling after Postmodernism* (2017). www.delloewenthal.com; www.safpac.co.uk.

What is Paranormal?

Some Implications for
Psychological Therapies

Edited by
Del Loewenthal

R Routledge
Taylor & Francis Group

LONDON AND NEW YORK

First published 2022
by Routledge
2 Park Square, Milton Park, Abingdon, Oxon OX14 4RN

and by Routledge
605 Third Avenue, New York, NY 10158

Routledge is an imprint of the Taylor & Francis Group, an informa business
Introduction and Chapter 7 © 2022 Del Loewenthal
Chapters 2–6 © 2022 Taylor & Francis
Chapter 1 © 2016 Andreas Sommer. Originally published as Open Access.

British Library Cataloguing in Publication Data
A catalogue record for this book is available from the British Library

ISBN: 978-1-032-03559-8 (hbk)
ISBN: 978-1-032-03566-6 (pbk)
ISBN: 978-1-003-18794-3 (ebk)

DOI: 10.4324/9781003187943

Typeset in Myriad Pro
by Newgen Publishing UK

Publisher's Note
The publisher accepts responsibility for any inconsistencies that may have arisen during the conversion of this book from journal articles to book chapters, namely the inclusion of journal terminology.

Disclaimer
Every effort has been made to contact copyright holders for their permission to reprint material in this book. The publishers would be grateful to hear from any copyright holder who is not here acknowledged and will undertake to rectify any errors or omissions in future editions of this book.

Contents

Citation Information

The following chapters were originally published in *European Journal of Psychotherapy and Counselling*, volume 18, issue 2 (2016). When citing this material, please use the original page numbering for each article, as follows:

Chapter 1

Are you afraid of the dark? Notes on the psychology of belief in histories of science and the occult
Andreas Sommer
European Journal of Psychotherapy and Counselling, volume 18, issue 2 (2016), pp. 105–122

Chapter 2

'They daren't tell people': therapists' experiences of working with clients who report anomalous experiences
Elizabeth C. Roxburgh and Rachel E. Evenden
European Journal of Psychotherapy and Counselling, volume 18, issue 2 (2016), pp. 123–141

Chapter 3

The paranormal as an unhelpful concept in psychotherapy and counselling research
Rose Cameron
European Journal of Psychotherapy and Counselling, volume 18, issue 2 (2016), pp. 142–155

Chapter 4

Phantom narratives and the uncanny in cultural life: psychic presences and their shadows
Samuel Kimbles
European Journal of Psychotherapy and Counselling, volume 18, issue 2 (2016), pp. 156–169

Chapter 5

Engaging the anomalous: reflections from the anthropology of the paranormal
Jack Hunter
European Journal of Psychotherapy and Counselling, volume 18, issue 2 (2016), pp. 170–178

Chapter 6

The client, the therapist and the paranormal: a response to the special edition on psychotherapy and the paranormal
Tony R. Lawrence
European Journal of Psychotherapy and Counselling, volume 18, issue 2 (2016), pp. 179–192

For any permission-related enquiries please visit:
www.tandfonline.com/page/help/permissions

Notes on Contributors

Rose Cameron, Counselling, Psychotherapy and Applied Social Science, University of Edinburgh, Edinburgh, Scotland, UK.

Rachel E. Evenden, Psychology Division, Centre for the Study of Anomalous Psychological Processes, University of Northampton, Northampton, England, UK.

Jack Hunter, Department of Archaeology and Anthropology, University of Bristol, England, UK.

Samuel Kimbles, C.G. Jung Institute of San Francisco, San Francisco, California, USA.

Tony R. Lawrence, Department of Psychology and Behavioural Sciences, Coventry University, Coventry, England, UK.

Del Loewenthal, University of Roehampton, UK; Southern Association for Psychotherapy and Counselling (SAFPAC), London, England, UK.

Elizabeth C. Roxburgh, Psychology Division, Centre for the Study of Anomalous Psychological Processes, University of Northampton, Northampton, England, UK.

Andreas Sommer, Churchill College & Department of History and Philosophy of Science, University of Cambridge, Cambridge, England, UK.

Introduction

What is paranormal: some implications for the psychological therapies?

Del Loewenthal

> "A layman will no doubt find it hard to understand how pathological disorders of the body and mind can be eliminated by 'mere' words. He will feel that he is being asked to believe in magic. And he will not be so very wrong for the words which we use in our everyday speech are nothing more than watered down magic." (Freud 1890: 285)

My thanks to Brottman for drawing my attention to the above quote and who in turn stated: "Although magic, symbol, and superstition are generally considered to be primitive forms of thinking, contemporary psychoanalysis is full of them" (2009: 471).

This book provides further developments of these ideas.

Whilst writing this introduction I went to examine a Doctorate in Psychotherapy and Counselling. As I started to go up the stairs to the university room used for such vivas the person coming down asked, pleasantly but firmly, if I would mind going back down 'so we don't pass on the stairs'. Was this an example of widespread belief in the paranormal? The doctorate itself was awarded, but it was an empirical study. Had it been only the development of theory would it have failed as such non-evidence based scholarly writings previously considered academically appropriate could now be regarded as, at best, also paranormal?

The paranormal could be seen as being fundamental to the psychological therapies. Occasionally a writer, more often a psychoanalytic one, brings this potential to our attention but questions of science, evidence-based practice and so forth continue to dominate. Yet does this continue to lead to 'what's denied running even more wild'? Further, might the lessening of the paranormal be primarily what is lost, the aura, through the increase in internet therapy (Risq 2020). This book reopens the question of the paranormal and the psychological therapies which continues not to go away, not only for psychoanalysis but the psychological therapies in general.

So, what is meant by the term 'paranormal'? For more than some, 'paranormal' is when there is not a scientific explanation. Indeed, Google's dictionary, as provided by Oxford Languages', definition is: 'denoting events or phenomena such as telekinesis or clairvoyance that are beyond the scope of normal scientific understanding'. This might lead to at least four further questions, the first being 'what is normal', the second 'what is taken as science?', the third, 'how do we distinguish this from pseudo-science?', the fourth, 'are the psychological therapies more an art than a science?'

> And what, if anything, has the paranormal to do with psychological therapists' interests in such concepts as the uncanny (Freud 1919), synchronicity (Jung 1960), the transpersonal (Daniels 2005; Mintz & Schmeidler 1983), telepathy (Totton 2003), mindfulness (Clarke 2014) and anomalous experiences (for example Sollod 1992)? There is indeed still occasionally, albeit minority, an interest in for example the ideas of Abraham and Torok (1994) as their
> '...creepier and darker metaphorics brings to life beings like the crypt, ghosts, goblins, and phantoms' for reinvigorating 'traditional Freudian psychoanalysis by shifting its metaphorical register to a rubric with a more occult sensibility.' (Glazier 2021)

This claim to return to exploring the paranormal, albeit, as with Freud, through attempting to call psychoanalysis a science, can be seen in the exploration by Frosh (2012) of hauntings (also see Fisher 2014 on 'hauntology'):

> '... psychoanalysis is also an active process of using the mechanisms of haunting. Much of this has to do with what is communicated at a spatial or temporal distance, whether between people who have no obvious physical connection to one another, or across generations ...... Much of the scholarship and clinical writing that has attended to this ... dimension of haunting has been concerned with the intergenerational transmission of trauma... But it has other elements too, to which Freud was attuned, notably questions of the generational continuity of ethnic and religious identity. In more contemporary language, it is also what underpins much postcolonial critique: how the societies of today carry with them the active ghosts of previous times. How does this happen, how is something not-known-about nevertheless passed on, sometimes to the extent that it is obviously re-enacted? More mysteriously still, is there something in the 'it is' of the present that is already reaching forward to the 'it will be' to come?' (Frosh 2012: 242)

In our current culture, we seem to have become obsessed with very narrow notions of evidence-based practice, where for example, randomised controlled trials (RCTs) are spoken of as the gold standard. Yet, RCTs in the case of psychological therapies can be seen as more a form of ritual magic covering up both their scientific absurdity and that we are unable to have an appropriate scientific approach to evaluating the therapies.

Another question is, will we one day have an appropriate science as indeed Freud had hoped? A related contribution to this argument was given in the seminal work of Roth and Fonagy's *What Works for Whom?* (2006), where they point out that just because there isn't the scientific evidence available for a particular approach, this doesn't mean to say that it isn't necessarily effective. Indeed, the intellectual roots of those who want to exclude any practice that is not RCT evidence-based can be seen to:

> '...lie in the Enlightenment and its ideals of reason, materialism and reductionism. ...that is, the belief that the only evidence for truth is just what can be measured by our observational means and technological resources.' (Heaton 2001: 239)

So, should we be saying that those psychological therapists and clients/patients who take part in practices that do not lend themselves to the magical thinking of RCT-type voodoo, believe in the paranormal? What place if any in psychotherapy is there for tradition, custom, intuition and love (Heaton 2001)?

Also how open can we as psychotherapists be to not knowing (Kokoli 2017; Cayne and Loewenthal 2006) without being over concerned, to the extent of a reaction formation, that we are not scientific but occult practitioners?

What then should be the 'normal' practices of psychological therapies? I have previously been fond of quoting Merleau-Ponty (2002 [1962]) who suggests that sometimes if we attempt to take away the mystery, we take away the thing itself. Elsewhere I have often done the equivalent of retweeting Emmanuel Levinas' (1961) argument that we should *accept* people, rather than attempt, the potential violence of, trying to *know* them. This last point has some similarity with Carl Rogers' (1957) notion of stressing the importance of the therapist's non-judgmental acceptance of the client. Furthermore, some of those, for example Laplanche (1989), who are interested in theory nevertheless warn us against filling in what we don't know with, for example, simple transference interpretations that no longer leave open other possibilities. Interestingly, as Borch-Jacobsen (1988) points out, the word 'transference' refers to a trance state. There is also a question whether such concepts as phenomenology are helpful here in keeping open possibilities and where they too end up unhelpfully 'filling in what we don't know'.

So, a scientific underpinning of the notion of paranormal as a basis for evidence-based practice might classify Merleau-Ponty (2002 [1962]), Levinas (1961), let alone Kristeva's subversive trinity of 'madness, holiness and poetry' (1984), as perhaps at best being 'paranormal'.

I recently attended a christening where, to my amazement, people I thought I had known for many years were crossing themselves, splashing themselves with water, and seemingly unquestioningly speaking of keeping Satan at bay. Should I now reconsider these people as paranormal, if not psychiatric?

However, to return to the consulting room, we may see a client who experiences sexuality in every encounter, which might be there but the rest of us 'normally' repress it. There again, this client may be imagining that we are asking him or her to carry out specific sexual acts which therapeutically, one might, for example, see more as a type of projection by the client. I find myself writing the above two sentences as if I can more readily accept the first sentence as a possibility, that is, something that is actually happening, whereas the second sentence, as a delusion of the client/patient. Yet how do I know any of this? Why do I not just accept that both may be beyond my and others' explanations and just term them as part of the paranormal? To take a final example: a client states that anything she does that gives her pleasure will lead to punishment, even to the extent that to speak of this to another could lead to something terrible happening to, in this instance, her therapist. How much am I able to enter the possibility that this is not just her experience but true? Could it be that it's beyond my cause and effect thinking that I fill in this case with regarding her magical thinking was a way that the client as a child attempted to safeguard herself against something that actually happened, or she imagined happened?

It is questions such as these that I hope this book will help open up in our increasingly 'evidence-based' suffocating world, where research would seem to have less and less to do with thoughtful practice. I am grateful to our contributors, published respondents and to Nick Totton and Edith Steffen who introduced me to some of them in what I hope will open up new possibilities for our practices. I also want to acknowledge the invaluable assistance I received in preparing what is now this book from Evrinomy Avdi, Betty Bertrand, Christian Buckland, Anastasios Gaitanidis, Elizabeth Nichol, Jay Watts and David Winter.

Chapter 1 is entitled 'Are you afraid of the dark? Notes on the psychology of belief in histories of science and the occult'. Here, the author Andreas Sommer offers a contribution to the debate concerning the tensions between 'rational' science, with particular reference to scientific psychology and the occult, and the roots of these tensions in the development of modern scientific practice. These tensions are placed within a cultural and historical context which provides an insight into why popular understandings of the 'conflict between science and the occult' still prevail.

In Chapter 2, "They daren't tell people': therapists' experiences of working with clients who report anomalous experiences', Elizabeth Roxburgh and Rachel Evenden present a qualitative study in which themes were derived from participants' interviews using an inductive thematic analysis. The findings show that clients were considered apprehensive about disclosing anomalous experiences due to fears about how these might be interpreted and in particular being stigmatised as having mental health issues.

Chapter 3 is by Rose Cameron on 'The paranormal as an unhelpful concept in psychotherapy and counselling research'. The author argues for a phenomenological rather than 'scientific' perspective on phenomena in psychotherapy and counselling that might be labelled as paranormal with particular reference to an episode from the author's therapeutic practice. In this chapter, a certain view is implied from the start by the author, in that, the paranormal can be considered as an obtrusive notion within psychotherapy.

Chapter 4 is by Samuel Kimbles and is entitled 'Phantom narratives and the uncanny in cultural life: psychic presences and their shadows'. In this paper, the author makes a strong case for examining the unconscious or 'phantom' dynamics that shape our attitudes, emphasising the importance of the collective experience through 'Cultural Complexes'. The author puts forward the idea of intergenerational transmission of traumatic group experiences that generate cultural complexes which subsequently, in turn, haunt the individual members of the group in the form of phantomatic experiences and narratives.

We then have our two published responses. The first one, Chapter 5, is by Jack Hunter and is entitled 'Engaging the anomalous: reflections from the anthropology of the paranormal'. Jack's paper provides us with a useful history of anthropological perspectives into the 'paranormal', pointing out that anomalous experiences are not limited to 'primitive' cultures but nevertheless they appear to be taboo within Euro-American academia. The author then draws implications of this for psychotherapy.

The second response, Chapter 6, is from Tony Lawrence who in his chapter 'The client, the therapist and the paranormal: a response' both critically and personally engages with the topic. Tony argues that taking a phenomenological stance is crucial for the therapist–client relationship when working with clients' presentations of ostensibly paranormal and anomalous experiences.

Finally, Chapter 7 'The magic of the relational' by Del Loewenthal puts the case for what we may regard as paranormal being the essence of the psychological therapies. The notion of relational therapy would appear to be of growing interest to counsellors, psychotherapists and psychoanalysts across all modalities. What though seems important is that there is something in 'the relational' which we can't fully name. Certain teachers as with psychological therapists have it more and whilst training schools attempt to bring it out in all, we never really know what that 'it' is. For some it's relationality, for others it's inter-subjectivity or tacit knowledge, or transference/countertransference or phenomenological and so forth. None seem fully adequate to explain what it is we experience in what might be called 'the between'. Whatever 'it' is, it does though seem to fit Google's Oxford dictionaries definition of the paranormal as 'denoting events or phenomena... that are beyond the scope of normal scientific understanding'. Yet, whilst psychoanalysis may be attempting more ways to name 'it', isn't relational magic there in every psychological therapy?

I just prefer to call it 'the magic of the relational'.

Occasionally a psychological therapist writes that such paranormal phenomena have relevance for the fields of both psychotherapy and psychoanalysis. To give another example Lazar (2001) in the consideration of non-verbal communication and mutual influence between therapist and patient. The hope is that this book is a further opportunity for any psychological therapist (counsellor, psychotherapist, psychoanalyst, psychologist, arts and play therapist, and so forth) to reconsider what relevance paranormal events and phenomena may have for their practices whatever their modality. Indeed, perhaps the chapters in this book will help readers consider the implications of regarding such 'unscientific' works, or even evidence-based practice or more importantly their and their clients' experiences, as vitally paranormal.

References

Abraham, N., and Torok, M. (1994). *The Shell and the Kernel: Renewals of Psychoanalysis, Vol. 1*. Rand, N. T. (ed.). Chicago: University of Chicago Press.

Borch-Jacobsen, M. (1988). *The Freudian Subject*. Redwood City, CA: Stanford University Press.

Brottman, M. (2009). Psychoanalysis and Magic: Then and Now. *American Imago*, 66(4), 471–489.

Cayne, J. and Loewenthal, D. (2006). 'Exploring the Unknown in Psychotherapy through Phenomenological Research'. *In:* Loewenthal, D. and Winter, D. (eds) *What is Psychotherapeutic Research?*, London: Karnac, pp. 117–132.

Clarke, I. (2014). The Perils of Being Porous: A Psychological View of Spirit Possession and Non-dogmatic Ways of Helping. *Self & Society*, 41(4), 44–49.

Daniels, M. (2005). *Shadow, Self, Spirit: Essays in Transpersonal Psychology*. Exeter: Imprint Academic.

Fisher, M. (2014). *Ghosts of My Life: Writings on Depression, Hauntology, and Lost Futures*. Alresford: Zero Books.

Freud, S. (1890). `Psychical (or Mental) Treatment'. *The Standard Edition of the Complete Psychological Works of Sigmund Freud Volume XVII (1917–1919): An Infantile Neurosis and Other Works*, London: Hogarth Press, pp. 283–302.

Freud, S. (1919). The 'Uncanny'. *The Standard Edition of the Complete Psychological Works of Sigmund Freud Volume XVII (1917–1919): An Infantile Neurosis and Other Works*, pp. 217–256.

Frosh, S. (2012). Hauntings: Psychoanalysis and Ghostly Transmission. *American Imago*, 69(2), 241–264. https://doi:10.1353/aim.2012.0009.

Glazier, W. (2021). Here Lies... Hermetics, Psychoanalysis, and Ethnocentrism: Using Abraham and Torok to Help Explain the Rise of Reactionary Social Groups. *Psychotherapy and Politics International*. https://doi.org/10.1002/ppi.1575.

Heaton, J. (2001). Evidence and Psychotherapy. *European Journal of Psychotherapy & Counselling*, 4(2), 237–248, https://doi:10.1080/13642530110080998.

Jung, C. G. (1960). *Synchronicity: An Acausal Connecting Principle*. Princeton, NJ: Bollingen Series, Princeton University Press.

Kokoli, A. (2017). 'An Extreme Tolerance for the Unknown: Art, Psychoanalysis and the Politics of the Occult'. *In:* Kokoli, A. (ed.) *In Focus: From the Freud Museum 1991–6 by Susan Hiller*. London: Tate Research Publication. *Available at:* www.tate.org.uk/research/publications/in-focus/from-the-freud-museum-susan-hiller/psychoanalysis-occult Accessed: 18 July 2021.

Kristeva, J. (1984). *Revolution in Poetic Language*. New York: Columbia University Press.

Laplanche, J. (1989). *New Foundations for Psychoanalysis*. Hoboken, NJ: Wiley-Blackwell.

Lazar, S. (2001). Knowing, Influencing, and Healing: Paranormal Phenomena and Implications for Psychoanalysis and Psychotherapy. February 2001. *Psychoanalytic Inquiry* 21(1), 113–131.

Levinas, E. (1961). *Totality and Infinity: An Essay on Exteriority*. Pittsburgh, PA: Duquesne University Press.

Merleau-Ponty, M. (2002[1962]). *Phenomenology of Perception*. London: Routledge.

Mintz, E. E. and Schmeidler, G. R. (1983). *The Psychic Thread: Paranormal and Transpersonal Aspects of Psychotherapy*. New York, N.Y: Human Sciences Press.

Rizq, R. (2020). What have we lost?, *Psychodynamic Practice*, 26(4), 336–344.

Rogers, C. R. (1957). 'The Necessary and Sufficient Conditions of Therapeutic Personality Change'. *In:* Kirschenbaum, H. and Henderson, V. L. (eds) *The Carl Rogers Reader, 1990*. London: Constable, pp. 219–235.

Roth, A. and Fonagy, P. (2006). *What Works for Whom? A Critical Review of Psychotherapy Research* New York: The Guilford Press.

Sollod, R. (1992). 'Psychotherapy with Anomalous Experiences'. *In:* R. Laibow, R. Sollod and J. Wilson (eds) *Current Perspectives on Anomalous Experiences and Trauma*. Dobbs Ferry, NY: Treat Publications, pp. 247–260

Totton, N. (2003). *Psychoanalysis and the Paranormal: Lands of Darkness*, Abingdon: Routledge.

Are you afraid of the dark? Notes on the psychology of belief in histories of science and the occult

Andreas Sommer

ABSTRACT

The popular view of the inherent conflict between science and the occult has been rendered obsolete by recent advances in the history of science. Yet, these historiographical revisions have gone unnoticed in the public understanding of science and public education at large. Particularly, reconstructions of the formation of modern psychology and its links to psychical research can show that the standard view of the latter as motivated by metaphysical bias fails to stand up to scrutiny. After highlighting certain basic methodological maxims shared by psychotherapists and historians, I will try to counterbalance simplistic claims of a 'need to believe' as a precondition of scientific open-mindedness regarding the occurrence of parapsychological phenomena by discussing instances revealing a presumably widespread 'will to disbelieve' in the occult. I shall argue that generalized psychological explanations are only helpful in our understanding of history if we apply them in a symmetrical manner.

Angst vor der Dunkelheit? Anmerkungen zur Psychologie des Glaubens in der Geschichte der Wissenschaft und des Okkulten

Infolge der neuesten Fortschritte innerhalb der Wissenschaftsgeschichte gilt der bis dato gängige Blick auf den inhärenten Konflikt zwischen Wissenschaft und dem Okkulten als hinfällig. Diese Neuerungen innerhalb der Wissenschaft wurden jedoch von der Öffentlichkeit nicht wahrgenommen. Insbesondere die Rekonstruktion der Genese der modernen Psychologie und ihren Verbindungen zu parapsychologischen Forschungen zeigen, dass sich letztere nicht einfach als Ausdruck von metaphysischer Voreingenommenheit verstehen lassen. Um nun einen Ausgleich zu schaffen, werde ich Fälle eines 'Willens zum Unglauben' diskutieren und davon ausgehend den Vorschlag machen, dass allgemeine psychologische Erklärungen nur dann hilfreich für ein Geschichtsverständnis sind, wenn wir sie in einer symmetrischen Art und Weise anwenden.

Tiene usted miedo a la oscuridad? Notas en la psicología de las creencias en historias acerca de la ciencia y lo oculto

La visión popular del conflicto inherente entre la ciencia y lo oculto, ha quedado obsoleta debido a los avances recientes en la historia de la ciencia. Sin embargo, estas revisiones historiográficas han pasado casi desapercibidas en la comprensión pública de la ciencia y la educación. Particularmente las reconstrucciones de la formación de la psicología moderna y sus conexiones con la investigación psíquica, nos muestran que la visión común de esta última, motivada por sesgos metafísicos no pasa la prueba de la realidad. En este artículo discuto ejemplos de una "voluntad de incredulidad" para contrabalancear las demandas simplistas de una "necesidad de creer" como precondición de una apertura científica de la mente en relación con la incidencia de fenómenos parapsicológicos, y sugiero que las explicaciones psicológicas generalizadas son útiles solamente en nuestra comprensión de la historia si las aplicamos de manera simétrica.

Hai paura del buio? Note sulla psicologia delle credenze nella storia della scienza e dell'occulto

La rappresentazione popolare della contrapposizione tra scienza e occulto è stata resa obsoleta dai recenti progressi della storia della scienza. Eppure, queste revisioni storiografiche sono state trascurate dalla conoscenza comune sulla scienza e dall'istruzione pubblica in generale. In particolare la ricostruzione di come si sia formata la psicologia moderna e dei suoi collegamenti con la ricerca psicologica dimostra una visione standardizzata di questi ultimi, giustificata da pregiudizi metafisici che non reggono la verifica. Per controbilanciare affermazioni semplicistiche relative a un 'bisogno di credere' come precondizione di una scientifica apertura mentale relativa all'insorgenza di fenomeni parapsicologici, discuto le istanze della 'volontà di credere' e suggeriscono che le spiegazioni psicologiche generiche sono utili alla nostra comprensione della storia solamente se le usiamo in modo bilanciato.

Avez-vous peur du noir ? Notes sur la psychologie de la croyance dans l'histoire de la science et l'histoire de l'occulte

L'opinion populaire concernant le conflit intrinsèque entre la science et l'occulte a été rendue obsolète par les récentes avancées de l'histoire des sciences. Pourtant ces révisions historiographiques sont passées inaperçues de la compréhension publique de la science et de l'éducation publique dans son ensemble. Les reconstructions de l'évolution de la psychologie moderne et de ses liens avec la recherche psychique peuvent montrer en particulier que la vision standard de cette dernière en tant que motivée par un bais métaphysique échoue à résister à son examen. Pour contrebalancer l'argument simpliste d'un 'besoin de croire' comme précondition à l'ouverture d'esprit scientifique concernant l'occurrence des phénomènes parapsychologiques, des exemples sont ici discutés de 'volonté de ne pas croire' et il est suggéré que des explications psychologiques généralisées sont seulement utiles pour nous aider à comprendre l'histoire à condition de les appliquer de manière symétrique.

Φοβάσαι το σκοτάδι; Σημειώσεις σχετικά με την ψυχολογία της πίστης στην ιστορία της επιστήμης και του μεταφυσικού

Η δημοφιλής άποψη της εγγενούς σύγκρουσης μεταξύ της επιστήμης και του μεταφυσικού έχει καταστεί παρωχημένη από τις πρόσφατες εξελίξεις στην ιστορία της επιστήμης. Ωστόσο, αυτές οι ιστοριογραφικές αναθεωρήσεις έχουν περάσει απαρατήρητες στη δημόσια κατανόηση της επιστήμης και της δημόσιας εκπαίδευσης γενικότερα. Οι ιδιαίτερες ανακατασκευές της διαμόρφωσης της σύγχρονης ψυχολογίας και η σύνδεσή της με την ψυχική έρευνα μπορούν να καταδείξουν ότι η κανονική οπτική της τελευταίας ως κινούμενης από την μεταφυσική προκατάληψη αποτυγχάνει να αντέξει τον λεπτομερή έλεγχο. Προκειμένου να αντισταθμίσω απλοϊκές αξιώσεις μιας «ανάγκης να πιστέψουμε» ως προϋπόθεση της επιστημονικής ευρύτητας του πνεύματος όσον αφορά την εμφάνιση των παραψυχολογικών φαινομένων, θα συζητήσω τις περιπτώσεις της «θέλησης να δυσπιστήσουμε» και δείχνω ότι οι γενικευμένες ψυχολογικές εξηγήσεις είναι χρήσιμες μόνο στην κατανόηση της ιστορίας αν εφαρμόζονται με συμμετρικό τρόπο.

'Ways of being in the world' in historical research and the therapeutic setting

At first glance, psychotherapists and historians appear to have very little in common. To be sure, both professions are concerned with human beings, but your clients are obviously alive, while my historical protagonists are long gone. The persons you work with usually seek you out to get help understanding and changing their individual present, whereas I select my historical actors in the hope they might prove useful to me as a lens to understand collective pasts. You empower your clients to become active collaborators in the therapeutic process by encouraging them to mobilize own resources, while my historical actors are perfectly at my mercy should I chose to distort their lives to make them fit any preconceived narratives of mine. Not least, your clients are protected by basic human rights and can take legal steps if they feel mistreated, whereas I have nothing to fear in consequence of, say, retroactively tainting a historical protagonist's reputation as the dead are unable to sue.

Yet, it seems that in a crucial sense some of these differences actually indicate a mutual work ethos. I take it for granted that the first step in establishing a fruitful client-therapist relationship requires the therapist's commitment to treat those seeking help on their own terms. Rather than forcing your own way of being in the world upon persons in your care, you will strive to base therapeutic interventions on a thorough understanding of where each is coming from. Ideally, historians are trained to observe very similar methodological maxims. For our job is no longer to justify the present by limiting reconstructions of the past through compatibilities with today's epistemological and metaphysical standards, but to faithfully resurrect the past by doing our best to obtain a thorough understanding of sentiments and existential categories that were actually at the disposal of the individuals whose ways of being in the world we aim to investigate.

Quite often, I struggle to get my head around beliefs and sentiments of my historical actors, even if I know this doesn't necessarily require me to drastically modify my own presuppositions and cultural conditionings. I expect similar issues to arise as challenges to therapeutic practice. A client may, for instance, report a certain class of recurring 'weird' experiences, such as fulfilled prophetic dreams of accidents and deaths, possibly intrusive telepathic rapport with a parent or lover they are in the process of separating from, frightening out-of-body experiences, visual or auditory hallucinations of dead relatives and friends, or dramatic 'poltergeist'-style episodes involving loud noises, levitating objects, and other 'things that go bump' in their homes or maybe even workplaces. In many cases, you may find it advisable not to encourage your client's belief in the reality of the reported phenomena, while trying to establish what emotional conflicts and issues each experience may represent.

On the other hand, you might have encountered instances where ostensibly 'paranormal' experiences, rather than being inherently unsettling, on the contrary inspired a client's confidence in higher and ultimately benevolent realities. Far from persuading such clients to abandon these apparently irrational and naive beliefs, you may have come to acknowledge that at least some individuals can exploit profound forms of 'transpersonal' optimism as highly effective means to cope with, and possibly even overcome, concrete hardships and emotional problems. And from conversations with various therapists I'm practically certain that there are cases where a client's fear of being considered 'not normal' or mentally ill simply by virtue of having such experiences constitute a major obstacle to therapeutic progress. After all, most of us were brought up in the belief that science has conclusively shown that these things are impossible, and that something must be wrong with those reporting experiences that appear to suggest otherwise.

Obviously, as a historian, I have no intention let alone competence to argue for the existence or non-existence of parapsychological (or 'psi') phenomena. It is merely as a potential token of assistance with such cases – however small it will be – the present article is written. In a sense, it could be viewed as complementary to recent clinical studies and revisions appearing to show that, whatever their ultimate nature, exceptional or 'paranormal' experiences are neither particularly uncommon nor intrinsically pathological (cf. Cardeña, Lynn, & Krippner, 2014). In fact, some of the recent historical research I shall try to distil in the following pages has revealed that the 'occult' was always a part of our scientific and intellectual heritage.

Science as a candle in the dark?

Unless you have had striking experiences of a seemingly occult nature yourself, you're probably not likely to believe that 'psi' phenomena occur. But even if you do, you probably know that it is wise to keep that belief to yourself if you expect your peers to view you as sane, critical and scientifically minded. And supposing you're a sceptic, you demand that belief should depend on sound empirical evidence, because the more outlandish a proposition the stronger the evidence must be to support it. But there simply is no scientific evidence, because wouldn't we all know if there was? For science, we have been brought up to believe, is intrinsically self-correcting and always on the lookout for anomalies that might bring about revolutionary scientific breakthroughs. Moreover, the very essence of scientific practice securing its self-correcting nature are intellectual core virtues – impartial love of truth, open-mindedness paired with discerning rigour, courageous anti-dogmatism and other qualities without which the scientific enterprise would quickly lose its appeal as intrinsically progressive and good.

Those holding this quasi-teleological view of scientific progress are also likely to believe the study of the history of science and medicine is irrelevant: if science always provides the most reliable mirror of reality, its past can constitute little more than a graveyard of errors and obsolete ideas. For many, the only story worthwhile telling is in the style of that modern bible of popular science, Carl Sagan's *The Demon-Haunted World: Science as Candle in the Dark* (Sagan, 1995). In fact, subsequent celebrity scientists with a metaphysical axe to grind like Neil deGrasse Tyson and Bill Nye in the US, and Richard Dawkins and Brian Cox here in Britain, have closely adhered to this standard way of preaching to the masses the gospel of science as a grand master narrative of humanity's journey from the deplorable, oppressive superstitions of the past towards the inherently liberating and humanistic (Western) sciences of the present.

Science popularizers laudably hammer home the message that science deserves that name only if it is firmly rooted in the intellectual virtues mentioned above, and if it strictly builds on the best available evidence. Curiously, however, these basic principles – which obviously should guide historical research no less than science – are nearly always dropped as soon as the question of the relationship between science and religion (the supposed breeding ground of occult belief) is concerned. Instead of systematic, impartial research, we find claims of their perennial incompatibility endlessly recycled in the mass media and the 'public understanding of science', while academic historical scholarship showing that the so-called conflict thesis of science and religion is largely a historiographical artefact stemming from the nineteenth century is simply ignored.

In fact, the popular notion of the supposedly self-evident opposition of science and religion – each routinely portrayed as monolithic entities epitomizing eternally progressive vs. regressive mindsets – turns out to be little more than a caricature, as soon as their interactions are reconstructed within original contexts and by paying attention to local, political, ideological and other factors usually passed over in triumphalist chronologies of progress (see, e.g. Brooke, 1991; Dixon, Cantor, & Pumfrey, 2010; Numbers, 2009).[1] Like any other human endeavour, science is not practiced in a cultural, political and metaphysical vacuum, and it is these 'extra-scientific' conditions of the past that have profoundly shaped scientific institutions, methods, research questions, and theories up the present. Recent studies in the history of neuroscience, for example, have revealed that contrary to present-day popular beliefs, epiphemonenalist standard views are no unequivocal corollary of neuroscientific advances. The view that the brain produces the mind has always been just one among various pre-existing metaphysical presuppositions, for which the modern mind and brain sciences have served as vehicles (Hagner, 1992, 2012; Harrington, 1987; Smith, 1992; Vidal, 2009; Weidman, 1999; Young, 1970).

A related myth is the view of the inherent opposition of scientific psychology and the occult. Contrary to ongoing attempts to demarcate modern psychology from parapsychology through simplistic historical assertions of the latter's intrinsic unscientificity (e.g. Ash, Gundlach, & Sturm, 2010; Marshall & Wendt, 1980), a clear-cut distinction has been difficult if not impossible to draw in terms of research, methods and representatives. This is particularly true for the infancy of professionalized psychology: Between 1889 and about 1909, investigations into 'marvellous' phenomena associated with mesmerism and spiritualism were discussed on important platforms of early academic psychology like the International Congresses of Psychology, which were initiated and organized by parapsychological researchers such as Charles Richet, Julian Ochorowicz, Arthur T. and Frederic W. H. Myers, Henry and Eleanor M. Sidgwick, and Albert von Schrenck-Notzing. 'Founding fathers' of the psychological profession, such as William James in the US and Théodore Flournoy in Switzerland, were active psychical researchers and attempted an integration of radical empirical parapsychological studies into fledgling psychology, while others, such as Théodule Ribot in France, appeared supportive of such attempts (Brower, 2010; Le Maléfan & Sommer, 2015; Plas, 2012; Shamdasani, 1994; Sommer, 2013a, 2013b; Taylor,

1985). Also flying in the face of assertions that scientific psychology had done away with the occult is the continuity of open-minded scientific interest in parapsychological phenomena within and beyond the psychological profession (Mauskopf & McVaugh, 1980; Sommer, 2013a, 2014b; Valentine, 2012).

Wills to believe

> He who believes in it carries out experiments in sorcery, and he who does not believe in it as a rule does not. But since man is known to have a great tendency to find confirmed what he believes in, and to this end might even apply a great ingenuity to deceive himself, to me the success of such experiments only proves that those conducting them believe in them to begin with. (Wundt, 1892, pp. 9–10)[2]

> The true opposites of belief, psychologically considered, are doubt and inquiry, not disbelief. (James, 1889, p. 322)

To say that the occult entanglements of modern psychology, and the sciences in general, have been squarely written out of public and disciplinary history is certainly not an overly melodramatic statement.[3] Interestingly, an axiom underlying the traditional historiography of science and the occult that has been obscuringing these links boils down to a psychological rather than historical explanation of open-minded scientific interest in occult phenomena, and a surprisingly simplistic one at that: metaphysical bias and an infantile 'need to believe' in transcendental realities.

The above quote by Wilhelm Wundt, the 'father' of professionalized psychology in Germany, shows that generalizing psychological explanations for scientific interest in 'paranormal' phenomena by an unhealthy obsession with the marvellous are not exactly new. In the US, Joseph Jastrow had launched his long career as self-appointed border-guard and popularizer of American psychology by proclaiming that open-minded scientific tests of the reported phenomena of spiritualism indicated a 'state of mind that is to be prevented' since it was 'dangerous to mental sanity' and 'morbidly hungry for something unusual, something mystic, something occult' (Jastrow, 1887, p. 8). A refusal to dismiss the occult was so dangerous for Jastrow and other opponents of psychical research 'because this system goes deeper, and appeals to the feelings, that it blinds its adherents to sense and reasoning' (loc. cit.). Much later, Edwin Boring, the eminent historian of experimental psychology, likewise insisted that it was 'quite clear that interest in parapsychology has been maintained by faith. People want to believe in an occult something' (Boring, 1966, p. xvi).

Unproblematic as such statements may seem at first glance, unfortunately the matter is not quite as straightforward. For once, we cannot simply assume that the remarkable outrage expressed by critics like Wundt, Jastrow and other hardliners in the fight against the 'occult' during the making of modern psychology was scientifically justified. Again and again, writing in their function as scientists, these critics in fact mainly relied on appeals to assumed social, cultural and not least religious dangers of a belief in 'occult' phenomena. Eschewing constructive dialogues with their targets of attack, opponents offered little dispassionate and constructive methodological critiques and favoured popular magazines and pamphlets rather than formal scholarly channels to get their polemics across. Epistemological positions, methods, aims and arguments of psychical researchers were misrepresented by reliance on generalized allegations of fraud and insinuations of methodological incompetence, the latter being tacitly explained through claims of metaphysical bias (Sommer, 2012, 2013a, Chapter 4; Taylor, 1996).

Moreover, by the late nineteenth century, any empirical approach to marvellous events had already been repudiated from intellectual discourse for over a century. Again contrary to widespread assumptions, however, it was predominantly political, philosophical and religious concerns rather than scientific work that had made fashionable the Enlightenment notion of belief in preternatural occurrences as an indicator of intellectual, moral and spiritual vulgarity at best, and mental illness at worst (cf. Cameron, 2010; Daston & Park, 1998; Porter, 1999; Sommer, 2013a, Chapter 1). Later, popularizers of professional psychology merely continued an overwhelmingly polemical war, relying on an Enlightenment standard rhetoric using fuzzy but immensely loaded terms such as 'mysticism', 'superstition', 'sorcery', 'enthusiasm' and similar catchwords to discredit intellectual interest in alleged occult phenomena. This strategy served to construct a public image of the 'new psychology' particularly in the US and Germany as inherently progressive and unified, and not least as practically useful in the combat of the supposed social and cultural dangers of spiritualism and other 'epidemic delusions' (Coon, 1992; Leary, 1987; Sommer, 2012).

Another stubborn myth regarding psychical research is that it has always been a reactionary movement, owing its existence to a childish reluctance to accept the self-evident truth of scientific materialism. While the history of scientific materialism itself thoroughly refutes the teleological standard narrative of materialism as a science-based and therefore obligatory worldview (Gregory, 1977; Lange, 1876–1877), not a few leading representatives of psychical research like its doyens in France (Charles Richet), Germany (Albert von Schrenck-Notzing), Poland (Julian Ochorowicz) and Italy (Enrico Morselli and Cesare Lombroso) have either been card-carrying materialists or positivists advocating a distinctively secular and anti-spiritualist psychical research (Brancaccio, 2014; Sommer, 2013a, Chapter 2, 2014a). To complicate matters further, we would be hard pressed to identify a single representative of scientific materialism among the early vocal psychological opponents of psychical research (cf. Hatfield, 1995). Not least, a continued openness to extra-sensory perception (ESP) within a distinctively materialist tradition, Freudian psychoanalysis (Devereux, 1974; Gyimesi, 2012; Totton, 2003), should make us sceptical of the psychical research vs. materialism stereotype. Yet, unchecked simplistic arguments from metaphysical bias that fail to stand up to historical scrutiny continue to be advanced even in professional philosophical discussions of parapsychology and the demarcation problem (Sommer, 2014a).

To simplify an immensely complicated story: the professionalization and beginning secularization of the sciences in the late nineteenth century occurred in an atmosphere that was marked by a vehement hostility not so much to religion but to 'magical thinking'. Scientific secularization and the rise of positivism were driven not by a materialist worldview, but mainly by rationalist and predominantly anti-clerical religious thinkers, who more often than not were just as programmatically opposed to materialism as they were to spiritualism and related large-scale occult movements of the time.

The opposition to magical thinking also crystallized in rather dramatic political events. The birth of modern experimental psychology in Germany, for example, occurred at the end of Bismarck's *Kulturkampf*. This was a national war against the Catholic church fought throughout the 1870s, which, after the March Revolution in 1848, could be called the German version of the French Revolution. Propagating an Enlightenment-style anti-'superstition' rhetoric, the *Kulturkampf* was vocally supported by leading popularizers of secularized science such as the outspoken anti-materialist Rudolf Virchow and the materialist Ernst Haeckel, who were both strictly unsympathetic to a radical empirical approach to the phenomena of spiritualism and mesmerism. The crucial thing to understand here is that opposition to investigations of the phenomena of mesmerism and spiritualism came from multiple and often mutually antagonistic camps. To say this was a climate not exactly conducive to parapsychological experimentation would therefore be an understatement.

When viewed in its original context, the aggressive opposition by early psychologists such as Wundt and Jastrow to unorthodox scientific activities appears to make sense in terms of a strategic imperative to protect the public image of nascent psychology from dangerous associations with the occult. The strange story of the coinage of the term 'Parapsychologie' by Max Dessoir also lends itself to an interpretation along these lines. Following attacks by Wundt and other leaders of the new psychological profession, Dessoir, a young psychologist who had initially tried to expand the methodological scope of German psychological experimentation in the late 1880s through an integration of parapsychological research, promptly embarked on a much safer career as a self-appointed guardian of rationality and *Volksaufklärer* (Sommer, 2013b).

But does political calculus and career opportunism really suffice to account for the ongoing bias in the public historiography of science and the occult? Although instances of violent opposition to new ideas is a commonplace in the history even of orthodox sciences, I cannot help but being struck by the persistent vehemence, the often hateful and emotional nature of some of the attacks that continue to inform this historiography.[4] I find myself essentially in agreement with psychoanalyst William Gillespie and many others, who observed that there was a strong tendency among critics to respond to the data of psychical research 'in an irrational, emotionally determined way' (Gillespie, 1956, p. 209). In fact, while sweepingly accusing elite psychical researchers of a regressive and undisciplined 'will to believe', critics have at the same time displayed strong indications of various fears. The American neurologist George M. Beard, for example, was not exactly a model of a rational and calm response to spiritualism and its impartial investigation, when he recommended that for 'logical, well-trained, truth-loving minds, the only security against spiritism is in hiding or running away' (Beard, 1879, p. 73). When Wundt was challenged to justify his dismissal of the experimental evidence presented by eminent German physicists in support of the reality of some of the phenomena of spiritualism, his fears of a downfall of modern culture and religion following in the train of a radical empiricism apparently got the better of his scientific curiosity, for he proclaimed:

> The moral barbarism produced in its time by the belief in witchcraft would have been precisely the same, if there had been real witches. *We can therefore leave the question entirely alone, whether or not you have ground to believe in the spiritualistic phenomena.* (Wundt, 1879, p. 592, my italics)

In France, the physicist Léon Foucault opposed investigations of table moving by exclaiming:

> If I saw a straw moved by the action of my will … I should be terrified. If the influence of mind upon matter does not cease at the surface of the skin, there is no safety left in the world for anyone (quoted in Sudre, 1960, p. 33).

Now I don't want to appear as trying to substitute one crude psychological explanation ('interest in occult phenomena has been motivated by an irrational need to believe', etc.) with another, equally simplistic one ('opposition to psychical research has been motivated by irrational fears') and use it as a historiographical argument. At the same time, once we acknowledge that cultural and personal biases constitute fundamental problems in any realm of human activity, the insight that we have to deal with them somehow seems inescapable. In the philosophy of science, the problem of incommensurability as formulated by writers like Thomas Kuhn and Paul Feyerabend already boils down to a squarely psychological one. Kuhn's own thoughts on instances of dogmatism throughout the history of science, for example, cautiously drew on psychological experiments in cognitive dissonance (Kuhn, 1996, esp. pp. 63–65, 112–115 and Chapter 10). Kuhn's ideas were also informed by the notion of 'absolute presuppositions' as discussed by the philosopher Robin Collingwood (1948). In the Kuhnian sense, these are fundamental propositions which scientists cannot afford to question or investigate but simply have to take for granted, such as the concept of causality, and the very possibility to get at fundamental truth in the first place.

This of course is the rationalist's arch dilemma, which we also find at the heart of the pragmatist conception of truth. After stating that some of our most

fundamental knowledge comes second hand and from unquestioned authorities, William James observed:

> Our belief in truth itself, for instance, that there is a truth, and that our minds and
> it are made for each other, – what is it but a passionate affirmation of desire, in
> which our social system backs us up? (James, 1897, p. 9).

For James, a radical empirical psychology of belief was forced to acknowledge
the tautological or self-confirming nature and foundation of much supposedly
rational belief. In the final analysis, it was passion rather than reason that James
found decided metaphysical positions and their rationalizations: Like anybody
else, the philosopher consciously or unconsciously wants to be the world a
certain way. It was his inevitable will to believe that

> loads the evidence for him one way or the other, making for a more sentimental or
> a more hard-hearted view of the universe, just as this fact or that principle would.
> He *trusts* his temperament. Wanting a universe that suits it, he believes in any rep-
> resentation of the universe that does suit it (James, 1907, p. 7, original emphasis).

With James I should concede that a compartmentalization of mentalities into
'tough-minded' or rational vs. 'tender-minded' or sentimental ways of being
in the world (or, as I would like to suggest adding, 'Platonic' vs. 'Epicurean') is
'indeed monstrously over-simplified and rude' (James, 1907, p. 35). But if we
grant a near infinite variability of mixtures existing between these tempera-
mental poles, it might serve some analytical purpose after all – particularly, if we
are to get at possible reasons for the immense public appeal of the indefinitely
more monstrously crude stereotypes regarding science, religion and the occult.

Indeed, James' reflections on the inevitably irrational origins of belief may
be as radical as Léon Foucault's above expression of horror in the face of a psychokinetically moved straw is consequent. Superficially perceived, Foucault's
quote may have a paranoid or comical ring to it. But I think philosopher Stephen
Braude has a point when he maintains that 'it's a very small step conceptu-
ally from psychokinetically nudging a matchstick to psychokinetically causing
someone to drop dead, or causing a car to crash' (Braude, 2007, p. 30).[5] Such
fears, according to Braude, might go a long way accounting for the often emotional off-hand dismissal of empirical indications in support of psi phenomena.
Moreover, a psychoanalytic truism has it that most of us simply don't want to
know the innermost contents of our minds. If this is the case, how likely are we
to welcome the prospect of others potentially having access? There might be
good reasons why psi researchers have not only considered the fear of psi as a
political problem, but also occasionally addressed it as a methodological issue
(e.g. LeShan, 1966; Tart, 1984; Tart & LaBore, 1986).

Lastly, the 'will to disbelieve' in magical powers and correspondences may
well be as old as the will to believe in them (cf. Whitmarsh, 2016). Philosopher
Michael Grosso (1990, pp. 244–246) reminds us that the ancient Greek materialist
philosophers Epicurus and Lucretius have been revered like messiahs by their
disciples for liberating them of the fear of evil magic, capricious gods and spirits,

and not least the horrifying uncertainty regarding the very nature of a hypothetical afterlife. Epiphenomenalism has always been a radical and convenient way to shut out these deep-seated existential fears, and to hold with authors like Otto Rank and Ernest Becker that the human desire for immortality was universal faces various problems. For once, Grosso argues that anthropologically and historically considered, the fear of death appears to be a relatively recent scourge of humankind, and might in fact be a main characteristic of modernity. With the anthropology of Sir James Frazer, Grosso also makes the interesting claim that fear *of the dead* is a much more promising universal than the fear of annihilation.[6]

At least a conscious antipathy towards the notion of immortality seems in fact fairly common. This has been suggested by the results of a survey on attitudes to immortality conducted by James' fellow pragmatist and psychical researcher, F.C.S. Schiller (1904). The philosopher Bernard Williams (Williams, 1976, Chapter 6) argued at length for the undesirability of immortality. C.D. Broad, who like James, Schiller and Henri Bergson was one of several philosophically distinguished presidents of the Society for Psychical Research, famously concluded his assessment of the empirical indications for post-mortem survival by stating that he should be 'slightly more annoyed than surprised' to find himself surviving bodily death (Broad, 1962, p. 430).

A more general confession of a will to disbelieve was made by another eminent philosopher, Thomas Nagel:

> Even without God, the idea of a natural sympathy between the deepest truths of nature and the deepest layers of the human mind, which can be exploited to allow gradual development of a truer and truer conception of reality, makes us more *at home* in the universe than is secularly comfortable. The thought that the relation between mind and the world is something fundamental makes many people in this day and age nervous. I believe this is one manifestation of a fear of religion which has large and often pernicious consequences for modern intellectual life (Nagel, 1997, p. 130, original italics).[7]

Finally, Hilary Putnam was comparatively vague when he stated that "Naturalism,' I believe, is often driven by fear, fear that accepting conceptual pluralism will let in the 'occult,' the 'supernatural'" (Putnam, 2004, p. 66).

For what it's worth, personally I find myself rather torn on the question whether magic and immortality are desirable. In my more introspective moments, I find Neoplatonic notions of a hidden interconnectedness of all living beings appealing, comforting and perhaps even conducive to mobilizing whatever little altruistic potential I might possess. On the other hand, the notion of other minds – incarnate as well as possibly discarnate – accidentally or intentionally snooping in the most intimate corners of my self, and having the power of manipulating and harming me through mere intentions, provokes a strong reaction of defence and unwillingness to grant the very possibility of transcendental correspondences. On a perhaps even more fundamental level, a part of me undoubtedly craves the kinds of social, aesthetic and intellectual fulfilments that life occasionally has to offer to continue indefinitely. But there are also moments when the prospect of a hypothetical impotence to end my existence if I wished so fills me with a feeling nothing short of a claustrophobic panic episode.

Conclusion

The study of the 'night side' of nature may induce a sense of wonder, but it is also inevitably appended with a whole range of fundamental fears – in addition to the above, we could adduce the fear of being duped, of a loss of control, and not least the fear of ridicule. Historian Peter Lamont (2013) has criticized the continued lumping together of all sorts of deviant beliefs in modern psychological scales supposing to measure 'paranormal belief'. There has been a wide spectrum of reasons for unorthodox beliefs over time, which psychologists are yet wont to ignore and sweepingly explain in terms of cognitive biases. With the psychology of paranormal belief continuing to thrive as a professional speciality, Lamont further notes a marked asymmetry in the complete absence of a tradition studying the psychology of paranormal *disbelief*. A similar asymmetry characterizes the public use of history in the continuing war against 'superstition', 'irrationality' and 'pseudoscience'.

Immanuel Kant famously stated that the essence of Enlightenment thought was the abolishment of dogmatism and false authorities, supplanted by the cultivation of courage to think for ourselves, his motto being *sapere aude!* – dare to know! Kant's appeal to intellectual courage necessarily admits fear. To radically think independently and question all authority is a scary thing indeed. But Kant himself did not follow his own principles when he responded to reports of ghostly goings-on with ridicule and armchair pathologization (Kant, 1900), an attitude that characterized the age of Enlightenment as much as undoubted advances in the cultivation of tolerance in other matters. The complimentary bogeys that plagued Kant and many of his contemporaries – the fear of materialism on the one hand, and of 'enthusiasm' (i.e. irrationality and 'superstition') on the other – continued throughout the nineteenth century and guided the professionalization of modern sciences.

The quasi-apocalyptic fears of supposed global dangers of magical belief that were so typical of the nineteenth century have not borne out, and in the face of recent historical studies documenting the integral role of continued occult mentalities in the making of modernity (cf. Albanese, 2007; Mannherz, 2012; Owen, 2004; Treitel, 2004), undiscriminating claims of a disenchantment of the world, let alone of the intrinsic backwardness and perilousness of occult beliefs, seem no longer feasible. But even though the original mentalities at work in the repudiation of radical empirical approaches to the occult may have vanished from public awareness, academic curricula still rest on epistemic prescriptions informed by these anxieties.

I might do worse than conclude these initial and somewhat crude observations with an appeal made by William James over a century ago: 'We all, scientists and non-scientists, live on some inclined plane of credulity. The plane tips one way in one man, another way in another; and may he whose plane tips in no way be the first to cast a stone' (James, 1897, p. 320). Some will no doubt misread this quote, along with my incomplete account of James' pragmatist analysis of the psychology of belief above, as a call to a disastrous epistemic and scientific anarchism and relativism. But like James I prefer to say that a frank acknowledgement of the rationalist dilemma must not be confused with an excuse for lazy thinking and arrogant dogmatism. Far from paralysing our critical faculties, its admission might on the contrary motivate us to try harder than ever to identify, accept and eliminate inevitable biases standing in the way of our cultivating benevolent open-mindedness coupled with 'never-sleeping suspicion of sources of error' (James, 1897, p. 303).

Notes

1. Some new age writers have also twisted the history of science to fit their own agendas. For a critique, see Brooke and Cantor (1998, Chapter 3).
2. My translation.
3. Regarding public history, see, for example, the hair-raisingly biased Wikipedia entries on parapsychology and psychical research.
4. These have been documented en masse not only by unorthodox scientists but also by supposedly impartial historians and sociologists of science. For pertinent literature, see, for example, Sommer (2014a).
5. Regarding popular beliefs in the efficacy of prayer and healing intentions, Braude also remarks that 'No process can be used only for the good. So, if we open the door to the salutary (or simply benign) effects of our thoughts on the external world, we must also open it to the destructive influence of our thoughts' (loc. cit.).
6. While Grosso equates fears of the unknown with fears of the shadow in the Jungian sense, Jung himself resorted to anthropological arguments when he took issue with the 'widespread bias' against well-documented parapsychological phenomena, which to him revealed 'all the symptoms of the primitive fear of ghosts', for 'even educated people who should know better occasionally utilize the most nonsensical arguments', and may even 'sign séance minutes and subsequently withdraw, as has been the case more than once, their signature, since what they had observed and verified was, as it were, impossible – as if one knew exactly what was possible!' (Moser, 1950, p. 11, my translation).
7. On the question of theistic religion, Nagel continues: 'I speak from experience, being strongly subject to this fear myself: I want atheism to be true and am made uneasy by the fact that some of the most intelligent and well-informed people believe in God and, naturally, hope that I'm right in my belief. It's that I hope there is not God! I don't want there to be a God; I don't want the universe to be like that' (loc. cit).

Acknowledgement

I am grateful for the support of a junior research fellowship at Churchill College, Cambridge.

Funding

This work was supported by a Wellcome Trust medical humanities doctoral studentship (grant no. 089723/Z/09/Z).

References

Albanese, C. L. (2007). *A republic of mind and spirit. A cultural history of American metaphysical religion*. New Haven, CT: Yale University Press.

Ash, M. G., Gundlach, H., & Sturm, T. (2010). Irreducible mind? *American Journal of Psychology, 123*, 246–250.

Beard, G. M. (1879). The psychology of spiritism. *North American Review, 129*, 65–80.

Boring, E. G. (1966). Introduction. Paranormal phenomena: Evidence, specification, and chance. In C. E. Hansel (Ed.), *ESP. A scientific evaluation* (pp. xiii–xxi). London: McGibbon & Kee.

Brancaccio, M. T. (2014). Enrico Morselli's *psychology of "spiritism"*: Psychiatry, psychology and psychical research in Italy around 1900. *Studies in History and Philosophy of Biological and Biomedical Sciences, 48*, 75–84.

Braude, S. E. (2007). *The gold leaf lady and other parapsychological investigations*. Chicago, IL: University of Chicago Press.

Broad, C. D. (1962). *Lectures on psychical research. Incorporating the perrott lectures given in Cambridge University in 1959 and 1960*. London: Routledge & Kegan Paul.

Brooke, J. H. (1991). *Science and religion. Some historical perspectives*. Cambridge: Cambridge University Press.

Brooke, J. H., & Cantor, G. (1998). *Reconstructing nature. The engagement of science and religion*. Edinburgh: T&T Clark.

Brower, M. B. (2010). *Unruly spirits. The science of psychic phenomena in modern France*. Urbana: University of Illinois Press.

Cameron, E. K. (2010). *Enchanted Europe: Superstition, reason, and religion, 1250–1750*. Oxford: Oxford University Press.

Cardeña, E., Lynn, S. J., & Krippner, S. (Eds.). (2014). *Varieties of anomalous experience: Examining the scientific evidence* (2nd ed.). Washington, DC: American Psychological Association.

Collingwood, R. G. (1948). *An essay on metaphysics*. Oxford: Clarendon Press.

Coon, D. J. (1992). Testing the limits of sense and science. American experimental psychologists combat spiritualism. *American Psychologist, 47*, 143–151.

Daston, L., & Park, K. (1998). *Wonders and the order of nature, 1150–1750*. New York, NY: Zone Books.

Devereux, G. (Ed.). (1974). *Psychoanalysis and the occult*. London: Souvenir Press.

Dixon, T., Cantor, G., & Pumfrey, S. (Eds.). (2010). *Science and religion. New historical perspectives*. Cambridge: Cambridge University Press.

Gillespie, W. H. (1956). Experiences suggestive of paranormal cognition in the psychoanalytic situation. In G. E. W. Wolstenhome & E. C. Millar (Eds.), *Ciba Foundation symposium on extrasensory perception* (pp. 204–214). London: Churchill.

Gregory, F. (1977). *Scientific materialism in nineteenth century Germany*. Dordrecht: Springer.

Grosso, M. (1990). Fear of life after death. In G. Doore (Ed.), *What survives? Contemporary explorations of life after death* (pp. 241–254). Los Angeles, CA: Tarcher.

Gyimesi, J. (2012). Sándor Ferenczi and the problem of telepathy. *History of the Human Sciences, 25*, 131–148.

Hagner, M. (1992). The soul and the brain between anatomy and *Naturphilosophie* in the early nineteenth century. *Medical History, 36*, 1–33.

Hagner, M. (2012). The electrical excitability of the brain: Toward the emergence of an experiment. *Journal of the History of the Neurosciences, 21*, 237–249.

Harrington, A. (1987). *Medicine, mind, and the double brain. A study in nineteenth-century thought*. Princeton, NJ: Princeton University Press.

Hatfield, G. (1995). Remaking the science of mind: Psychology as natural science. In C. Fox, R. Porter, & R. Wokler (Eds.), *Inventing human science: Eighteenth-century domains* (pp. 184–231). Berkeley: University of California Press.

James, W. (1889). The psychology of belief. *Mind, 14*, 321–352.

James, W. (1897). *The will to believe and other essays in popular philosophy*. London: Longmans, Green.

James, W. (1907). *Pragmatism: A new name for some old ways of thinking*. London: Longmans, Green.

Jastrow, J. (1887). Review of preliminary report of the Seybert Commission. *Science, 10*, 7–8.

Kant, I. (1900). *Dreams of a spirit-seer, illustrated by dreams of metaphysics*. (E. F. Goerwitz, Trans.). London: Sonnenschein & (original German publication in 1766).

Kuhn, T. S. (1996). *The structure of scientific revolutions* (3rd ed.). Chicago, IL: University of Chicago Press.

Lamont, P. (2013). *Extraordinary beliefs. A historical approach to a psychological problem*. Cambridge: Cambridge University Press.

Lange, F. A. (1876–1877). *Geschichte des Materialismus und Kritik seiner Bedeutung in der Gegenwart* [History of materialism and critique of its present significance] (Vol. 2, 3rd ed.). Iserlohn: Baedeker.

Le Maléfan, P., & Sommer, A. (2015). Léon Marillier and the veridical hallucination in late-nineteenth and early-twentieth century French psychology and psychopathology. *History of Psychiatry, 26*, 418–432.

Leary, D. E. (1987). Telling likely stories: The rhetoric of the new psychology, 1880–1920. *Journal of the History of the Behavioral Sciences, 23*, 315–331.

LeShan, L. (1966). Some psychological hypotheses on the non-acceptance of parapsychology as a science. *International Journal of Parapsychology, 8*, 367–381.

Mannherz, J. (2012). *Modern occultism in late imperial Russia*. DeKalb: Northern Illinois University Press.

Marshall, M. E., & Wendt, R. A. (1980). Wilhelm Wundt, spiritism, and the assumptions of science. In W. G. Bringmann & R. D. Tweney (Eds.), *Wundt studies: A centennial collection* (pp. 158–175). Toronto: Hogrefe.

Mauskopf, S. H., & McVaugh, M. R. (1980). *The elusive science. Origins of experimental psychical research*. Baltimore, MD: Johns Hopkins University Press.

Moser, F. (1950). Vorrede [preface] by C. G. Jung. In *Spuk. Irrglaube oder Wahrglaube? Eine Frage der Menschheit* [Hauntings. Delusion or true belief? A question of mankind] (pp. 9–12). Baden: Gyr.

Nagel, T. (1997). Evolutionary naturalism and the fear of religion. In *The last word* (pp. 127–143). Oxford: Oxford University Press.

Numbers, R. L. (Ed.). (2009). *Galileo goes to jail and other myths about science and religion*. Cambridge, MA: Harvard University Press.

Owen, A. (2004). *The place of enchantment. British occultism and the culture of the modern*. Chicago, IL: University of Chicago Press.

Plas, R. (2012). Psychology and psychical research in France around the end of the 19th century. *History of the Human Sciences, 25*, 91–107.

Porter, R. (1999). Witchcraft and magic in enlightenment, romantic and liberal thought. In B. Ankarloo & S. Clark (Eds.), *Witchcraft and magic in Europe. The eighteenth and nineteenth centuries* (pp. 191–282). Philadelphia: University of Pennsylvania Press.

Putnam, H. (2004). The content and appeal of "naturalism". In M. De Caro & D. Macarthur (Eds.), *Naturalism in question* (pp. 59–79). Cambridge, MA: Harvard University Press.

Sagan, C. (1995). *The demon-haunted world: Science as a candle in the dark*. New York, NY: Random House.

Schiller, F. C. S. (1904). The answers to the American branch's questionnaire regarding human sentiment as to a future life. *Proceedings of the Society for Psychical Research, 18*, 416–453.

Shamdasani, S. (1994). Encountering Hélène: Théodore Flournoy and the genesis of subliminal psychology. In S. Shamdasani (Ed.), *Théodore Flournoy. From India to the planet mars: A case of multiple personality with imaginary languages* (pp. xi–li). Princeton, NJ: Princeton University Press.

Smith, R. (1992). *Inhibition: History and meaning in the sciences of mind and brain*. Berkeley: University of California Press.

Sommer, A. (2012). Psychical research and the origins of American psychology: Hugo Münsterberg, William James and Eusapia Palladino. *History of the Human Sciences, 25*, 23–44.

Sommer, A. (2013a). *Crossing the boundaries of mind and body. Psychical research and the origins of modern psychology* (Unpublished PhD thesis). London: University College London.

Sommer, A. (2013b). Normalizing the supernormal: The formation of the "Gesellschaft für Psychologische Forschung" ["Society for Psychological Research"], c. 1886–1890. *Journal of the History of the Behavioral Sciences, 49*, 18–44.

Sommer, A. (2014a). Psychical research in the history and philosophy of science. An introduction and review. *Studies in History and Philosophy of Biological and Biomedical Sciences, 48*, 38–45.

Sommer, A. (Ed.) (2014b). Psychical research in the history of science and medicine. Special section. *Studies in History and Philosophy of Biological and Biomedical Sciences, 48*, 38–111.

Sudre, R. (1960). *Treatise on parapsychology*. (C. E. Green, Trans.). London: Allen & Unwin.

Tart, C. T. (1984). Acknowledging and dealing with the fear of psi. *Journal of the American Society for Psychical Research, 78*, 133–143.

Tart, C. T., & LaBore, K. (1986). Attitudes toward strongly functioning psi: A preliminary study. *Journal of the American Society for Psychical Research, 80,* 163–173.

Taylor, E. (1985). Psychotherapy, Harvard, and the American Society for Psychical Research: 1884–1889. *Proceedings of presented papers: The Parapsychological Association, 28th annual convention* (pp. 319–346). Medford, MA: Tufts University.

Taylor, E. (1996). *William James: On consciousness beyond the margin.* Princeton, NJ: Princeton University Press.

Totton, N. (Ed.). (2003). *Psychoanalysis and the paranormal. Lands of darkness.* London: Karnac.

Treitel, C. (2004). *A science for the soul. Occultism and the genesis of the German modern.* Baltimore, MD: Johns Hopkins University Press.

Valentine, E. R. (Ed.). (2012). Relations between psychical research and academic psychology in Europe, the USA and Japan. Special issue, *History of the Human Sciences, 25* (2), 1–164.

Vidal, F. (2009). Brainhood, anthropological figure of modernity. *History of the Human Sciences, 22,* 5–36.

Weidman, N. N. (1999). *Constructing scientific psychology. Karl Lashley's mind–brain debates.* Cambridge: Cambridge University Press.

Whitmarsh, T. (2016). *Battling the gods: Atheism in the ancient world.* London: Faber & Faber.

Williams, B. (1976). *Problems of the self: Philosophical papers 1956–1972.* Cambridge: Cambridge University Press.

Wundt, W. (1879). Spiritualism as a scientific question. An open letter to professor Hermann Ulrici, of Halle. *Popular Science Monthly, 15,* 577–593.

Wundt, W. (1892). *Hypnotismus und Suggestion* [Hypnotism and suggestion]. Leipzig: Engelmann.

Young, R. M. (1970). *Mind, brain and adaptation in the nineteenth century.* New York, NY: Oxford University Press.

'They daren't tell people': therapists' experiences of working with clients who report anomalous experiences

Elizabeth C. Roxburgh and Rachel E. Evenden

ABSTRACT

Objectives. This study explored the experiences of therapists who have worked with clients reporting anomalous experiences (AEs) to consider how they addressed such issues in therapy sessions. An AE is defined as 'an uncommon experience (e.g. synesthesia) or one that, although it may be experienced by a significant number of persons (e.g. psi experiences), is believed to deviate from ordinary experience or from the usually accepted explanations of reality according to Western mainstream science'. *Method.* Semi-structured face-to-face interviews were conducted with eight therapists who had worked with at least one client who had reported an AE in therapy. An inductive thematic analysis was conducted on transcripts. *Results.* Four themes were derived from participants' data, which were labelled using short participant extracts: 'Testing the waters', 'Exploration not explanation', 'It's special but it's not unique' and 'Forewarned and forearmed'. *Conclusions.* Participants felt that clients were apprehensive about disclosure of AEs due to fears about how AEs might be interpreted. Findings highlight the importance of therapists exploring the meaning of AEs with clients, rather than imposing an explanation and having access to accurate and reliable information about AEs.

"Sie wagen es nicht anzusprechen": Erfahrungen von Therapeuten mit Klienten, die von anomalen Erlebnissen berichten

Ziele. Die Studie untersucht die Erfahrung von Therapeuten mit Klienten, die von anomalen Erlebnissen (AEs) berichteten und wie die Therapeuten in der Sitzung dieses Thema behandelten. Daraus werden Implikationen für die therapeutische Praxis und Ausbildung abgeleitet. Design. Die Studie basiert auf einer qualitativen Inhaltsanalyse teilstrukturierter Interviews. Darüber hinaus wurde auf Grundlage der Transkripte eine induktive Kategorienbildung vorgenommen. Methode. Es wurden teilstrukturierte 'face-to-face' Interviews mit acht Therapeuten erhoben, die mit mindestens einem AE-Klienten gearbeitet haben. Ergebnisse. Vier Kategorien konnten aus den vorhandenen Daten extrahiert werden: "Erst mal vorfühlen", "Erkunden nicht Erklären", "Es ist ungewöhnlich aber nicht besonders" sowie "Vorwarnen und Wappnen". Schlussfolgerungen. Die Studienteilnehmer nahmen die Klienten als besorgt wahr, wenn von diesen AEs offengelegt wurden. Dieses Gefühl resultiert aus dem gesellschaftlichen Stigma bei Themen zur psychischen Gesundheit sowie den Ängsten der Klienten, wie die AEs wohl von weiteren Teilen der Gesellschaft interpretiert werden. Die Ergebnisse unterstreichen die Bedeutung des Therapeuten und dessen Kompetenz, dem Sinn von AEs mit dem Klienten zusammen nachzuspüren und gleichzeitig verlässliche Informationen über AEs zu besitzen bereit zu stellen.

"No se atreven a decírselo a la gente": Experiencias de trabajo terapéutico con clientes que informan acerca de experiencias anormales (EAs)

Objetivos: El objetivo de este estudio fue explorar las experiencias de terapeutas que han trabajado con clientes con experiencias anómalas (EAs), para considerar cómo dichos clientes han confrontado estas experiencias en las sesiones y las implicaciones para la formación y la práctica terapéuticas. Diseño: Se utilizó un método cualitativo que implicó entrevistas semi-estructuradas y se realizó un análisis inductivo de las transcripciones. Método; se realizaron ocho entrevistas semi-estructuradas frente a frente con terapeutas que habían trabajado al menos con un cliente que informó acerca de EAs. Resultados: De los datos obtenidos se derivaron cuatro temas los cuales se etiquetaron por medio de frases cortas de los participantes: "probando la profundidad de las aguas", "exploración sin explicación", "es algo especial pero no único" y "advertido y precavido". Conclusiones: según los participantes, los clientes se mostraron aprehensivos acerca de comunicar sus EAs, lo cual se deriva del estigma relativo a aspectos de salud mental, así como también a los miedos de los clientes en relación a cómo la sociedad interpreta estos fenómenos. Los resultados destacan la importancia de la exploración por parte de los terapeutas, del significado de las EAs para los clientes y del acceso a una información fidedigna y confiable con relación a estas EAs.

'Ciò che non si osa dire alla gente': esperienze di terapeuti nel lavoro con clienti che riferiscono esperienze anomale

Obiettivi. Lo scopo di questo studio è esplorare le esperienze di terapeuti che hanno lavorato con clienti che hanno raccontato esperienze anomale (AE) prendendo in considerazione il modo in cui tali esperienze sono affrontate in terapia e le implicazioni per la pratica terapeutica e per il training. Disegno di ricerca. Si è scelto un approccio qualitativo che implica interviste semi-strutturate, sulle trascrizioni è stata condotta un'analisi tematica induttiva. Metodo. Interviste semi-strutturate face to face sono state condotte con otto terapisti che avevano lavorato con almeno un cliente che aveva riportato AE. Risultati. Quattro temi emergono dall'analisi dei dati e sono stati etichettati con brevi estratti dalle interviste: 'testare le acque', 'esplorazione non spiegazione', 'è speciale, ma non unico', e 'uomo avvisato, mezzo salvato'. Conclusioni. I partecipanti percepivano la preoccupazione dei clienti rispetto al comunicare AE, ciò derivava da uno stigma connesso a questioni di salute mentale, oltre ai timori dei clienti relativi a come le AE possano essere interpretate dalla società. I risultati sottolineano l'importanza che i terapisti esplorino con i clienti i significati attribuiti alle AE e abbiano accesso a informazioni accurate e affidabili su tali eventi.

'Ils n'osent pas en parler' : expérience des thérapeutes travaillant avec des clients qui rapportent des expériences anormales

Objectifs : Le but de cette étude était d'explorer les expériences des thérapeutes ayant travaillé avec des clients qui rapportent des expériences anormales (AEs) afin de voir comment ils ont géré de telles expériences en séance, les implications pour la pratique thérapeutique ainsi que pour la formation. Une AE est définie comme "une expérience peu commune (comme la synesthésie) ou qui, bien que vécue par un nombre significatif de personnes (comme les expériences relatives au psi), est considérée comme déviante par rapport à l'expérience ordinaire ou par rapport aux explications généralement acceptées de la réalité selon la vision de la science mainstream occidentale".

Design : Une approche qualitative a été choisie comportant des entretiens semi-directifs et une analyse des retranscriptions d'entretiens suivant une analyse thématique inductive.

Méthode : Des entretiens semi-directifs en face-à-face ont été menés auprès de huit thérapeutes ayant travaillé avec au moins un client qui avait fait état d'une AE.

Résultats : Quatre thèmes ont été établis à partir des données auxquels un titre a été donné en utilisant les termes des participants : `prendre le pouls', `exploration pas explication', `c'est spécial mais ce n'est pas unique' et `un homme averti en vaut deux'

Conclusions : Les participants ont eu le sentiment que leurs clients appréhendaient de dévoiler leurs AEs, ce qui semblait être le résultat d'une stigmatisation liée aux peurs qu'ils avaient quant à l'interprétation qui pourrait être faite des AEs par la société en général et par des cliniciens en particulier. Les résultats montrent qu'il est important pour les thérapeutes d'explorer la signification des AEs avec les clients, plutôt que d'en imposer une, et d'avoir accès à des informations précises et fiables concernant les AEs.

«Δεν τολμούν να πουν στους ανθρώπους»: οι εμπειρίες των θεραπευτών που εργάζονται με πελάτες που αναφέρουν ανώμαλες εμπειρίες

Στόχοι. Ο σκοπός αυτής της μελέτης ήταν να διερευνήσει τις εμπειρίες των θεραπευτών που έχουν εργαστεί με πελάτες που αναφέρουν ανώμαλες εμπειρίες (AE) για να εξετάσουν πώς θα αντιμετωπιστούν τέτοιες εμπειρίες σε θεραπευτικές συνεδρίες και τις συνέπειες για τη θεραπευτική πρακτική και την κατάρτιση. Σχεδιασμός. Μια ποιοτική προσέγγιση που εμπεριέχει ημι-δομημένες συνεντεύξεις και μια επαγωγική θεματική ανάλυση διεξήχθη στο απομαγνητοφωνημένο υλικό. Μέθοδος. Ημι-δομημένες πρόσωπο με πρόσωπο συνεντεύξεις με οκτώ θεραπευτές που είχαν εργαστεί με τουλάχιστον έναν πελάτη ο οποίος είχε αναφερθεί σε AE. Αποτελέσματα. Προέκυψαν τέσσερα θέματα από τα δεδομένα που είχαν επισημανθεί χρησιμοποιώντας τις σύντομες φράσεις: «Ελέγχοντας τα νερά», «Εξερεύνηση και όχι εξήγηση»,« Είναι ιδιαίτερο αλλά όχι μοναδικό», και «Προειδοποιημένος και προετοιμασμένος». Συμπεράσματα. Οι συμμετέχοντες θεώρησαν ότι οι πελάτες ήταν ανήσυχοι σχετικά με την εξωτερίκευση των AE και ότι αυτό προήλθε από το στίγμα που συνδέεται με τα προβλήματα ψυχικής υγείας, καθώς και τους φόβους του πελάτη σχετικά με το πώς οι AE μπορεί να ερμηνευθούν από την ευρύτερη κοινωνία. Τα ευρήματα υπογραμμίζουν τη σημασία της διερεύνησης από τους θεραπευτές της έννοιας των AE με τους πελάτες της πρόσβασής τους σε ακριβείς και αξιόπιστες πληροφορίες σχετικά με αυτές.

An anomalous experience (AE)[1] is defined as follows:

> an uncommon experience (e.g. synesthesia) or one that, although it may be experienced by a significant number of persons (e.g. psi experiences), is believed to deviate from ordinary experience or from the usually accepted explanations of reality according to Western mainstream science. (Cardeña, Lynn, & Krippner, 2014, p. 4)

Some of the AEs that have been reported in the literature include extrasensory perception (ESP), near-death experiences (NDEs), out-of-body experiences (OBEs), contact with the deceased and synchronicity experiences (SEs) (see Appendix 1). A substantial proportion of the general population claim to have had AEs, with a number of surveys reporting prevalence rates of over 50% (see Dein, 2012).

Given that some individuals find AEs distressing or have existential questions following the experience (Kramer, Bauer, & Hövelmann, 2012), therapists may reasonably expect to encounter clients who are seeking support or who want to explore the significance of the experience. In a survey with mental health professionals in The Netherlands, Eybrechts and Gerding (2012) found that 59% of respondents had been in contact with a client reporting problems associated with spirit contact, 55% with ESP and 51% with psychic healing. However, 83% had not taken part in any courses about these topics and 35% expressed a need for more training in this area. Likewise, research conducted on the prevalence and phenomenology of SEs, found that 44% of a sample of 226 therapists had experienced SEs in the therapeutic setting, but that these experiences came as a shock to therapists and challenged their concept of reality (Roxburgh, Ridgway, & Roe, 2015; Roxburgh Ridgway, & Roe, 2016). Similarly, focus groups with trainee counsellors have revealed that they do not feel equipped to work with clients reporting AEs and that they would benefit from learning about the different types of AEs that they could be presented with (Roxburgh & Evenden, submitted).

In Europe, mainly France, Germany and Holland, specialist counselling services have been set up for the specific purpose of counselling clients who report AEs (see Kramer et al., 2012) and some of these have furnished us with information about the different types of AEs that clients seek support for. For example, Belz and Fach (2012) at the Institut für Grenzgebiete der Psychologie und Psychohygiene (IGPP: Institute for Frontier Areas of Psychology and Mental Hygiene) in Germany found 53% of the 1465 cases recorded to be related to poltergeist and apparition phenomena, 41% to be related to ESP, 38% to be associated with internal presence and influence (e.g. spirit possession), 15% to be associated with external presence and nightmares (e.g. sleep paralysis), 10% to be related to SEs and 7% to be associated with mediumship.

In terms of supporting individuals who have had AEs, suggestions have been made about specific techniques and approaches that might be beneficial in work with clients, such as mapping a timeline to see if there is a correspondence between emotional life events and when AEs occur or adopting a Rogerian approach (Kramer, 2012), holotropic breathwork and hypnosis (Ahmed, 2012), dreamwork techniques (Krippner & Friedman, 2010), bibliography (Noble, 1987), psychoeducation, guided imagery and art therapy (Greyson, 1997), group therapy (Parra, 2012) and normalising and demythologising AEs (Bauer et al., 2012; Gerding, 2012). Guidelines have also been published offering advice on how to counsel individuals who have AEs (e.g. Hastings, 1983; Siegel, 1986). For example, Hastings outlines several steps that can be followed: (1) ask the person to describe the experience, (2) listen without judging, (3) reassure the person that they are not 'mad', (4) name the type of AE, (5) provide information about what is known about the AE, (6) develop reality tests to establish whether the AE is genuine and (7) address the psychological reactions that result from the AE. Although this would seem to offer some valuable recommendations based on basic counselling skills, psychoeducation and reality testing, it could be argued that this is too generic, but also that it is not the role of the therapist to establish the authenticity of AEs as in step six (Evrard, 2012; Parra, 2012). It also relies on therapists having knowledge about AE research and theories, in addition to existing counselling skills, so as to provide clients with sufficient information about the process they are going through, and to explain what is known about the phenomenon. Recent research suggests that this might not translate to practise, as when clients have disclosed AEs in mainstream therapeutic contexts, they have reported that they do not feel listened to, accepted or understood (Taylor, 2005), consider the help they receive as inadequate (Eybrechts & Gerding, 2012), fear being ridiculed or pathologised and are eager to explore the meaning of the experience with an open-minded therapist (Roxburgh & Evenden, in press).

Whilst the growing field of 'clinical parapsychology' is making some progress towards establishing theoretical, research and clinical material, including case studies, on how to deal with AEs in therapeutic settings (for an overview see Kramer et al., 2012), most of these endeavours have come from outside of the UK. There have been no studies, to the authors' knowledge, that have investigated how therapists have worked with clients reporting AEs in UK counselling services. In order to redress this gap in the counselling field, this study aims to explore the experiences of therapists who have worked with such clients to gain an insight into what they think would be useful when addressing AEs, whether they feel competent working with clients reporting AEs, and whether they have received specialist training incorporating AEs. As such, this research acknowledges the need to generate a better understanding of how therapists have worked with clients reporting AEs and whether they have found any approaches helpful or unhelpful so that findings can help inform better therapeutic practice.

Method

Design

A qualitative method was adopted to explore the experiences of therapists who have worked with clients reporting AEs. Thematic analysis was considered appropriate for our research aims as we were interested in whether there are any commonalities in the way therapists work with clients reporting AEs. It is also considered a useful approach 'when you are investigating an under-researched area, or with participants whose views on the topic are not known' (Braun & Clarke, 2006, p. 11). Ethical approval was obtained from the School of Social Sciences Ethics Committee at the authors' university and ethical guidelines of the British Association for Counselling and Psychotherapy (BACP) were adhered to.

Participants

Purposive sampling was used to recruit therapists who had worked with at least one client who had reported an AE. As part of a separate survey study investigating the range and incidence of AEs in a secular counselling setting over a 1-year period, information about the interview study was distributed to therapists at two charity organisations. We also circulated information about the research to therapists within our network of contacts. Sample size was determined by

Table 1. Participants' details.

Pseudonym	Gender	Length of time practising	AE reported by clients	Orientation	Interview duration (mins)
Walter	M	15	Synchronicity Sense of presence Unusual healing Psychic experiences	Integrative psychotherapist/bodywork therapist	48
Harriet	F	7	Sense of presence	Gestalt therapist/play therapist/CBT	45
Charlotte	F	5	Sense of presence Auras Apparitions/visions Unusual death-related experiences	Psychodynamic counsellor	50
Graham	M	16	Spirit possession Sense of presence Mediumship Witchcraft Poltergiest Spiritual crisis	Transpersonal psychotherapist	48
Diane	F	13	Sense of presence NDE Hauntings/apparition	Integrative counsellor	50
Penny	F	27	Synchronicity Sense of presence	Transpersonal psychotherapist/hypnotherapist	89
Lisa	F		Sense of presence	Transpersonal psychotherapist	48
Sally	F	4	Witchcraft Spirit possession	Integrative/transpersonal psychotherapist	33

a number of factors including access to participants, the richness of data and guidelines for conducting thematic analysis (Braun & Clarke, 2013). Eight therapists took part in the study and consisted of two males and six females. Length of time practising varied between 4 and 27 years ($M = 12$ years). Their therapeutic orientations included transpersonal, integrative, CBT, hypnotherapy, psychodynamic and Gestalt (Table 1). Pseudonyms have been assigned to protect the identity of the participants and any personally identifiable information has been changed or removed to ensure anonymity. Participants were not required to provide any personal details about clients.

Data collection

Semi-structured interviews were conducted by the second author at a time and place convenient to participants, which included the counselling service where they worked, a university room or their home. Interview questions were open-ended and non-leading and focused on how participants had worked with clients presenting with AEs, for example, 'Can you describe the most memorable AE that was reported by a client?', 'How did it make you feel?', 'What therapeutic

Table 2. Table of themes and meaning.

Theme	Meaning
'Testing the waters'	Client's fears around disclosure, distress more about fear of madness, feel as though they need to brush it under the carpet/deny aspects of self, disclosure risks diagnosis, stigma/societal barriers
'Exploration not explanation'	Interested in the meaning of the experience, client's perspective, therapist may have a theory but clients have their own perspective, important to explore how the client feels about the AE
'It's special but it's not unique'	Normalising the experience, human experience, AEs are common, might be comforting to the client, cultural awareness
'Forewarned and forearmed'	Normalise experiences in training/integrate into CPD/assimilation of knowledge, trainees need preparing. Need to be transparent about what we can support and refer on if necessary

approach(es) have you adopted?', 'How have such approaches been beneficial?', 'Have any approaches/techniques been unhelpful?', 'Did the experience affect how you worked with the client?' and 'What training did you receive on working with AEs?'. Participants had the option of reviewing the schedule before agreeing to take part in the study, but we highlighted that additional questions may be asked due to the semi-structured nature of the interview format. Duration of interviews varied between 33 and 89 min (Table 1).

Data analysis

An inductive thematic analysis was conducted on the interview data as outlined by Braun and Clarke (2006). In order to maximise the validity of themes both authors independently analysed the data and then came together to discuss and refine findings. The first stage in the analytical process consisted of both authors immersing themselves in the data, reading the transcripts several times and exploring their deeper meaning in terms of the implications for therapists and therapeutic practice. Any interesting observations about the narrative, in relation to the research questions, were noted on the transcripts and initial lists of potential themes were generated. Both authors then reviewed these lists and began a process of clustering themes in order to develop a final table of themes that accurately reflected repeated patterns of meaning within the data (Table 2). This data-driven form of analysis together with the semi-structured nature of the interview guide enabled participants to set their own parameters in terms of what they felt important to discuss, which enabled a more thorough understanding of the topic. Short participant extracts were used to name the themes.

Reflexive statement

Both authors are academics and BACP registered counsellors (with training in integrative approaches) who volunteer for charity organisations. In terms of our own experiences of working with clients who have reported AEs, we note the importance of respecting different explanatory models and to acknowledge the experience as subjectively real for the individual. As we were interested in therapists' experiences and perspectives, we did not aim to establish the veracity of AEs or theorise on the ontology of such experiences, and were mindful in the analysis to be objective and open-minded.

Findings

Four key themes were derived from participants' data: 'Testing the waters', 'Exploration not explanation', 'It's special but it's not unique' and 'Forewarned and forearmed'.

'Testing the waters'

When discussing their experiences of working with clients who had reported AEs, participants naturally drew attention to the client's experience and the manner in which they disclosed AEs. Participants talked about how clients are often hesitant to disclose that they have had an AE for fear that they will be seen as 'mad'. The consequences of this were that clients often 'tested the waters' before sharing details of AEs with therapists. With reference to clients who have sensed the presence of the deceased after bereavement, Charlotte states that they often see how she responds to such issues first before fully divulging the extent of their experiences, such as maintaining communication with deceased loved ones, or sometimes she can tell that they want to discuss an experience and need a bit of encouragement to do so:

> Nearly everybody I see for bereavement, I think, talks to the person they've lost, and some of them will tell you that straight away, others will take a little bit of prompting, because they think it means they're going mad ... I often find that people are quite, sort of tentative, you know, and see how I react to certain things (Charlotte)

Likewise, Diane reflected on how clients are seeking 'permission' that it is okay to talk about AEs in the therapy session without being seen as 'crazy':

> Some of them do pre-empt with 'You're gonna think I'm crazy when I tell you this' and they do look for a bit of reassurance, and ask me 'Does that fit with your belief system?' also when mentioning psychics as well ... they are saying 'Is this on our agenda? Can we visit this? Can I admit this?'. (Diane)

Participants also felt that there was still a lot of stigma attached to mental health issues in general which results in some clients being reluctant to seek support but that perhaps this applied even more so to clients who had AEs. Harriet believed that society's views about 'madness' and AEs becomes entrenched in clients, serving as a barrier to the therapeutic process, and that as a result clients felt that their experiences had to be 'brushed under the carpet':

Often, there's a big link with shame in some of these beliefs as well because I know of clients that actually say that they feel as if they daren't tell people because they'll be stigmatised, because people will think that they're mad or it's not rational or in their line of work they shouldn't be having these kind of thoughts or ways of being, so they kind of feel as if they have to be brushed under the carpet in some way or deny those aspects of themselves. (Harriet)

'Exploration not explanation'

In terms of working with clients who report AEs, the majority of participants pointed out that it was important to explore the meaning of the experience from the client's perspective, rather than impose their own interpretation. Harriet mentioned working in the 'here and now' to explore how the client felt about the experience:

> Opposed to staying with the, this happened and this is my explanation for it, is the, 'Well let's look at that and explore it. How did you arrive at that?' And I work very much in the here and now as well. So what's coming up for you when you think about that now? And so we can bring it into the session as well. So, say for example, if it was a client that said that they felt, I don't know, they felt that their dead husband was around them, I'd be saying, 'Do you have a sense that he's around you now, then? Tell me what that's like. And how is that helpful to you? When might it be less helpful?' You know, and so we'd work in that way (Harriet)

Charlotte added that she never discusses with clients whether AEs are genuine or not, reiterating that the essential therapeutic process is to explore what the experience means to the client as an individual, in contrast to making a judgement as to what is real or not or imposing one's own explanation:

> Some of them want to explore, you know, 'Do I think it is real?' 'What do I think its significance is?' Which, of course, I don't actually ever voice an opinion, and, but I try to find out what it means to them, and then go from there (Charlotte)

Similarly, Sally mentioned that she is interested in hearing the client's personal account and takes the AE at face value regardless of how implausible it may seem:

> I accept the story whatever it is, even if it's outlandish even if it rings like totally crazy to me and I try to gauge the capacity of the client. 'So what if this experience is true, what if someone's casting a spell on you, how do you think this is affecting you?', for example, and that's how I kind of try to understand their story (Sally)

Participants also emphasised that exploring the meaning of AEs is no different from how they would normally work. This is exemplified by Harriet and Diane who reflect on the process of therapy being the same for AEs as other issues:

> I don't find that working in this way is any different in some ways to working with the client who has experienced horrific, enduring abuse or the client that, I don't know, has an eating disorder, the client that self-harms. Because for me, the process of, is still very similar which is the, as I say, entering the client's world whilst still in your own world and exploring that and looking at

it from the client's perspective and then looking at integration or looking at finding places for things, or looking at letting things go, you know (Harriet)

I don't really adopt or use a specific approach except to explore it as I would anything else that they may have brought. To me it's just something else that they've experienced in their very interesting, complex, and complicated lives (Diane)

'It's special but it's not unique'

Participants reflected on how some clients find AEs special in some way, for example, they mentioned how clients who had sensed the presence of the deceased often find the experience therapeutic as it helped with the grieving process, but that at the same time clients also seek reassurance that they are not the only ones having AEs. As Lisa stated:

> I think because AEs are anomalous people do get ya know nervous or anxious, they do feel the need for reassurance, clients feel the need for reassurance when they see something that they know is not the norm. There is a need for, 'is this ok?' (Lisa)

They also reflected on how important it was to normalise the experience by letting clients know that other people have had similar experiences. Participants mentioned that this seemed to help ground clients as well as reassure them that it was safe to share their AEs, as Walter and Sally state:

> I'm amazed at how much things calm down when you encourage a person to befriend the process and also when you start saying look 'this has happened to other people, it's not about you, this is a, this is like a human experience' (Walter)

> As soon as the client understands that whatever they bring I'm not just gonna pass judgement or pass them off as crazy, or suggest they need medication or even 'I can't deal with this', as soon as they get this response they are more equipped to deal with this, that kind of somehow helps them and myself to place the experience back into a more kind of grounded and rationale context (Sally)

Participants also pointed out that in some cultures AEs are not viewed as anomalous and are routinely seen as a normal part of human experience:

> I realised in my mental health placement that there seems to be a lot of presence of ethnic minority so when you actually go and speak to clients about the issue of witchcraft it's not mad to them because where they grew up it's very normal and people do cast spells when they hate you so … it has somehow got out of control … but you know what if they find a therapist that knows about it and is capable of putting it back into the right frame whereas rather than say 'Oh my God that doesn't exist, that is crazy', so a cultural awareness is also very important (Sally)

> Within certain cultures, a lot of what we're exploring today would be absolutely embraced, you know, and my guess is that if there were counsellors within certain cultures, they wouldn't be saying, 'Oh no, we can't work with this in six sessions', they'd be, 'bring it in, let's have a look at it' (Harriet)

'Forewarned and forearmed'

Participants felt that it would better prepare therapists to work with clients who report AEs if trainee counsellors/psychotherapists were introduced to the topic early on in their training, emphasising the need for normalisation of AEs not only in society (as per theme 1) and the therapeutic session (as per theme 3), but also 'normalisation within the initial trainings' (Harriet). Graham felt that it would be useful to familiarise therapists with the concept of AEs because 'unless you have some real … erm … faith experience going on it can be rather difficult coz it can be rather daunting if you are faced with anything yourself'. He added that therapists should be aware of their own limits and be prepared to refer clients elsewhere if they felt that AEs were not something they felt comfortable working with:

> There is also things going on out there that is in the spiritual realms that if you're not prepared to deal with it then you need to have a very strong sign over your forehead saying 'look I don't do spiritual stuff' … you know take it to someone else down the road coz it frightens the hell out of me (laughs) (Graham)

Charlotte echoed the necessity of referring on, but also mentioned that therapists have a responsibility for educating themselves on issues that they are not familiar with:

> I think people should be aware, and, I mean, as I say, to me it's no different to anything else that comes up in counselling, that if you don't know enough about it, either go and find out, or if you can't find out or don't feel comfortable working with it, then you should find, you know, refer them on to somebody who does (Charlotte)

Diane used 'magpie' as a metaphor to represent the assimilative process of therapists continuing their own professional development with further workshops:

> We should be a discipline that attends workshops on things that look interesting, the phrase 'magpies' springs to mind. So we go around collecting lots of ideas up and putting them in the bag … I like to think that as a discipline we would magpie this into our own practice in some way (Diane)

Discussion

This study explored therapists experiences of working with clients who had reported AEs. One of the main findings was that participants felt clients had been reluctant to disclose AEs for fear of being seen as 'mad' and so they often 'tested the waters' to see how therapists would respond. Farber (2003) estimated that two-thirds of clients leave something unsaid during therapy sessions and that the most common problems are related to sexual issues, violence, abuse and feelings of failure. It remains to be seen how common it is for clients to withhold information about AEs but this finding suggests that it might be fruitful to explore this further. Farber adds that there are several factors that affect client disclosure including shame, not wanting to hurt their therapists, considering the issue unimportant or because the decision to not disclose may be a coping strategy. Participants in the current study believed that client apprehension around disclosure stemmed from stigma attached to mental health issues as well as client fears about how AEs might be interpreted by wider society. This finding corroborates research conducted by the authors that explored clients' experiences of seeking support for AEs, as participants in that study also mentioned testing the waters before sharing details of their experiences as well as a fear of being labelled with a mental disorder if they did (Roxburgh & Evenden, in press).

The findings from both of these studies on AEs draw attention to clients' motives for not seeking counselling and align with the proposition made by Vogel, Wester, and Larson (2007) that social stigma is one of the most significant factors why individuals may avoid seeking help. Alarmingly, they cite a study in which 90% of the sample agreed that fear of being seen as 'crazy' was a potential barrier to seeking help. In addition to social stigma, they also argue that treatment fears, fear of emotion, anticipated utility and risk and self-disclosure are other factors that cause individuals to evade counselling. Interestingly, they propose that different problems may elicit different avoidant responses, for example, treatment fears have been found to be associated with help-seeking for academic problems but not interpersonal or drug problems. Given the wide range of different types of AEs, it may be worthwhile if future research investigated whether there are any particular barriers or facilitators associated with seeking support for different types of AEs. One area of exploration that has received relatively little attention in the counselling literature is locus of control in relation to help-seeking behaviour. Applied to the topic of AEs this could, for example, explore whether individuals who report different types of AEs make different attributions about loci of causality, stability and controllability of their experiences (Weiner, 1974), and in turn if this affects whether they seek support or not. It might be that individuals who claim to experience haunting or alien abduction phenomena, for example, make external attributions (i.e. attribute the phenomena to an outside force or being) and do not seek support because of the anticipated utility and risk factor (i.e. they do not believe that therapy can help with their type of problem or experience).

In terms of the implications for practise, these findings highlight the necessity for therapists and therapeutic services to be active in countering the debilitating effects of stigma. For example, Corrigan and Penn (as cited in Vogel et al., 2007) argue that this can be achieved in three ways: protest (e.g. therapists should be vocal and draw attention to negative portrayals of mental health), education (e.g. providing accurate information about mental health) and contact (e.g. reaching out to those experiencing mental health issues or setting up support groups). In terms of AEs specifically, this could be achieved by therapists, services and training organisations having adequate and reliable information about AEs and the potential link with mental health (Dein, 2012), including research findings and case studies, but also peer-facilitated support groups for AEs, such as those set up by the hearing voice network for individuals who hear voices.

In addition, given that participants felt that clients are often seeking permission that it is okay to discuss AEs, therapists could directly ask about these experiences at the assessment stage, not unlike guidelines for working with religious/spiritual issues which suggest taking a spiritual history (see Moreira-Almeida, Koenig, & Lucchetti, 2014). However, further research is necessary to elicit clients' reactions to being directly asked about AEs as well as the impact of such experiences on the therapeutic process. With reference to broaching the subjects of race, ethnicity and culture during the counselling process, Day-Vines et al. (2007) identify a continuum of five different broaching styles that could potentially be applied to raising the subject of AEs: (1) avoidant (issues are rarely discussed or deemed important), (2) isolating (may ask a single question out of feeling obligated to address the subject at least once but the subject remains off-limits as a topic of counselling concern), (3) continuing/incongruent (may consider the subject but has limited skills to fully explore in a way that is empowering for the client), (4) integrated/congruent (therapists broach subjects effectively and have integrated this behaviour into their professional identity, it has become a part of their routine) and (5) infusing (broaching represents a way of being and a lifestyle choice). Whilst little is known about which style clients might prefer in relation to AEs, we do know that the avoidant and isolating styles would be considered as antithetic to the findings reported here as both clients (Roxburgh & Evenden, in press) and therapists feel it is important to be able to discuss AEs in therapy. Moreover, findings emphasise that hesitant disclosure or palpable non-disclosure on behalf of the client should be legitimate concerns for the therapist that need to be managed within the dyadic relationship, and that there may be cues in the session that can be picked up which reflect a testing of the water in order to encourage clients to discuss their AEs with less hesitancy.

Another notable finding was that participants felt it was important to explore the meaning of AEs with clients rather than impose an explanation or make a judgement as to the authenticity of such experiences. Again, this validates findings from research with clients who have sought support for AEs (Roxburgh & Evenden, in press) as participants in that study also mentioned the importance of being able to make sense of the experience with an open-minded therapist. It also confirms the view that it is not the therapist's role to establish the reality of AEs (Parra, 2012). Participants also noted that clients sought reassurance that they were not the only ones having AEs and that normalisation often alleviated clients' anxieties about this. We acknowledge that normalisation could potentially be problematic, due to the definition of AEs placing these experiences outside of ordinary experience or as deviating from the usually accepted explanations of reality according to Western mainstream science. However, the definition also recognises that AEs may be experienced by a significant number of people and thus normalisation could involve reassuring clients that they are not the only ones to have had such experiences. This would be similar to the guidelines recommended by Hastings (1983) in terms of naming the type of AE and discussing with the client what is known about the AE.

These findings are congruent with studies that have compared clinical and non-clinical samples to investigate predictors of distress associated with AEs, as normalising and validating contexts in which experiences can be accepted, understood and shared were shown to be associated with lower distress. Moreover, it has been argued that it is not necessarily the AE that causes psychological distress but rather individuals' appraisals of the experience as socially and culturally unacceptable (Brett, Heriot-Maitland, McGuire, & Peters, 2013; Heriot-Maitland, Knight, & Peters, 2012).

Participants said that they would work the same way with AEs as they would with any other client issue. This may be reassuring to other therapists, particularly trainees, who have not yet encountered a client reporting an AE or who have wondered how they might work with such issues (Roxburgh & Evenden, submitted). This finding resonates with the common factors model in psychotherapy which argues that therapeutic outcome is related to factors that all approaches share, such as the therapeutic relationship, rather than factors or techniques specific to particular approaches (Cooper, 2008). This is in contrast to recommendations made in clinical guidelines (e.g. by the National Institute for Health and Clinical Excellence) that therapists should use particular approaches with particular types of problems (e.g. CBT for depression) because they have been empirically supported. Given the paucity of research on AEs and therapeutic outcome, in contrast to the wealth of efficacy research on depression and anxiety, further research is needed to explore whether different types of AEs respond to different ways of working.

It is interesting that participants felt that there was a need for the topic of AEs to be introduced to therapists in their training programmes or for workshops to be available, given that they felt they would work with AEs in the same way as other issues. However, the suggestion seemed to stem more from the belief that therapists would benefit from hearing about the different types of AEs and associated research and theoretical material rather than being shown specific techniques for how to work with such experiences, which is a similar finding to research conducted on the training needs of therapists in relation to the issue of working with AEs (Roxburgh & Evenden, submitted). Participants felt that this would better prepare therapists to be aware of their 'comfort zone', but would also help them to be able to normalise such experiences by being able to reassure clients that others have also reported similar experiences, particularly in the case of clients sensing the presence of the deceased after bereavement, which all but one participant had worked with.

One of the limitations of this research was that only White European therapists came forward to be interviewed. Although some participants reflected on cultural differences with respect to how AEs may be understood, future research could explore the perspectives of a more diverse range of therapists. In addition, the majority of therapists in this sample worked in an integrative or transpersonal way and it may be that therapists from other orientations or professions would have different views about working with clients who report AEs. Indeed different practitioners have varied in terms of their explanations for AEs and how they respond to clients reporting AEs (Roxburgh et al., 2016; Eybrechts & Gerding, 2012). It is speculated that this may be due to differences in training and/or personal beliefs about the nature and causes of such issues, which could have implications for how AEs are addressed. Likewise, it would be useful to know whether specific types of AEs elicit different or similar views in therapists and what impact therapists own experiences of AEs might have on the therapeutic process.

Conclusion

Participants reflected on how clients are often reluctant to disclose AEs to them for fear of being seen as 'mad'. This validates findings from interviews with clients who have sought support for AEs as participants in that study (Roxburgh & Evenden, in press) also mentioned a fear of being pathologised. In terms of addressing AEs that clients have reported, participants emphasised the importance of exploring the meaning with clients rather than imposing an explanation or making a judgement as to the authenticity of AEs. They also said that they would work the same way with AEs as they would with other issues but that it might be useful for therapists to have reliable and accurate information about AEs and/or for trainees to be introduced to the topic whilst undertaking practitioner training.

Notes

1. We note that AEs are also sometimes referred to as exceptional human experiences, out of the ordinary experiences, paranormal experiences, or unusual experiences in the literature.
2. This list is not exhaustive and participants also mentioned working with clients reporting additional AEs such as auras, witchcraft, and spirit possession.

Funding

This work was supported by the Bial Foundation [grant number 108/12].

References

Ahmed, D. S. (2012). Psychotherapeutic approaches to major paranormal experiences (MPE). In W. H. Kramer, E. Bauer, & G. H. Hövelmann (Eds.), *Perspectives of clinical parapsychology: An introductory reader* (pp. 66–87). Bunnik: Stichting Het Johan Borgman Fonds.

Bauer, E., Belz, M., Fach, W., Fangmeier, R., Schupp-Ihle, C., & Wiedemer, A. (2012). Counseling at the IGPP – An overview. In W. H. Kramer, E. Bauer, & G. H. Hövelmann (Eds.), *Perspectives of clinical parapsychology: An introductory reader* (pp. 149–167). Bunnik: Stichting Het Johan Borgman Fonds.

Belz, M., & Fach, W. (2012). Theoretical reflections on counselling and therapy for individuals reporting ExE. In W. H. Kramer, E. Bauer, & G. H. Hövelmann (Eds.), *Perspectives of clinical parapsychology: An introductory reader* (pp. 168–189). Bunnik: Stichting Het Johan Borgman Fonds.

Braun, V., & Clarke, V. (2006). Using thematic analysis in psychology. *Qualitative Research in Psychology, 3*, 77–101.

Braun, V., & Clarke, V. (2013). *Successful qualitative research*. London: Sage.

Brett, C., Heriot-Maitland, C., McGuire, P., & Peters, E. (2013). Predictors of distress associated with psychotic-like anomalous experiences in clinical and non-clinical populations. *British Journal of Clinical Psychology, 53*, 213–227.

Cardeña, E., Lynn, S. J., & Krippner, S. (Eds.). (2014). *Varieties of anomalous experience: Examining the scientific evidence* (2nd ed.). Washington, DC: American Psychological Association.

Cooper, M. (2008). *Essential research findings in counselling and psychotherapy: The facts are friendly*. London: Sage.

Day-Vines, N. L., Wood, S. M., Grothaus, T., Craigen, L., Holman, A., Dotson-Blake, K., & Douglass, M. J. (2007). Broaching the subjects of race, ethnicity, and culture during the counseling process. *Journal of Counseling & Development, 85*, 401–409.

Dein, S. (2012). Mental health and the paranormal. *International Journal of Transpersonal Studies, 3*, 61–74.

Evrard, R. (2012). Clinical psychology of anomalous experiences: Roots and paradigms. In W. H. Kramer, E. Bauer, & G. H. Hövelmann (Eds.), *Perspectives of clinical parapsychology: An introductory reader* (pp. 89–105). Bunnik: Stichting Het Johan Borgman Fonds.

Eybrechts, M. V., & Gerding, J. L. F. (2012). Explorations in clinical parapsychology. In W. H. Kramer, E. Bauer, & G. H. Hövelmann (Eds.), Perspectives of clinical parapsychology: An introductory reader (pp. 35–48). Bunnik: Stichting Het Johan Borgman Fonds.

Farber, B. A. (2003). Patient self-disclosure: A review of the research. *Journal of Clinical Psychology, 59*, 589–600.

Gerding, J. L. F. (2012). Philosophical counselling as part of clinical parapsychology. In W. H. Kramer, E. Bauer, & G. H. Hövelmann (Eds.), *Perspectives of clinical parapsychology: An introductory reader* (pp. 103–117). Bunnik: Stichting Het Johan Borgman Fonds.

Greyson, B. (1997). The near-death experience as a focus of clinical attention. *Journal of Nervous Mental Disease, 185*, 327–334.

Hastings, A. (1983). A counseling approach to parapsychological experience. *Journal of Transpersonal Psychology, 15*, 143–167.

Heriot-Maitland, C., Knight, M., & Peters, E. (2012). A qualitative comparison of psychotic-like phenomena in clinical and non-clinical populations. *British Journal of Clinical Psychology, 51*, 37–53.

Kramer, W. H. (2012). Experiences with psi counselling in Holland. In W. H. Kramer, E. Bauer, & G. H. Hövelmann (Eds.), *Perspectives of clinical parapsychology: An introductory reader* (pp. 7–19). Bunnik: Stichting Het Johan Borgman Fonds.

Kramer, W., Bauer, E., & Hövelmann, G. (Eds.). (2012). *Perspectives of clinical parapsychology: An introductory reader.* Bunnik: Stichting Het Johan Borgman Fonds.

Krippner, S., & Friedman, H. L. (2010). *Debating psychic experience: Human potential or human illusion?.* New York, NY: Praeger.

Moreira-Almeida, A., Koenig, H. G., & Lucchetti, G. (2014). Clinical implications of spirituality to mental health: Review of evidence and practical guidelines. *Revista Brasileira Psiquiatria, 36*, 176–182.

Noble, K. D. (1987). Psychological health and the experience of transcendence. *The Counseling Psychologist, 15*, 601–614.

Parra, A. (2012). Group therapy approach to exceptional human experiences: An Argentinean experience. In W. H. Kramer, E. Bauer, & G. H. Hövelmann (Eds.), *Perspectives of clinical parapsychology: An introductory reader* (pp. 88–102). Bunnik: Stichting Het Johan Borgman Fonds.

Roxburgh, E. C., Ridgway, S., & Roe, C. A. (2015). Exploring the meaning in meaningful coincidences: An interpretative phenomenological analysis of synchronicity in therapy [Special Issue]. *European Journal of Psychotherapy and Counselling, 17*, 144–161.

Roxburgh, E. C., Ridgway, S., & Roe, C. A. (2016). Synchronicity in the therapeutic setting: A survey of practitioners. *Counselling and Psychotherapy Research, 16*, 44–53.

Roxburgh, E. C., & Evenden, R. E. (in press). Most people think you're a fruit loop: Clients' experiences of seeking support for anomalous experiences. *Counselling and Psychotherapy Research.*

Roxburgh, E. C., & Evenden, R. E. (submitted). It's about having exposure to this: Investigating the training needs of therapists in relation to the issue of anomalous experiences.

Siegel, C. (1986). Parapsychological counselling: Six patterns of response to spontaneous psychic experiences. In W. G. Roll (Ed.), *Research in parapsychology* (pp. 172–174). Metuchen, NJ: Scarecrow Press.

Taylor, S. F. (2005). Between the idea and the reality: A study of the counselling experiences of bereaved people who sense the presence of the deceased. *Counselling and Psychotherapy Research, 5*, 53–61.

Vogel, D. L., Wester, S. R., & Larson, L. M. (2007). Avoidance of counseling: Psychological factors that inhibit seeking help. *Journal of Counseling & Development, 85*, 410–422.

Weiner, B. (1974). *Achievement motivation and attribution theory.* Morristown, NJ: General Learning Press.

Appendix 1. List of AEs used in the research[2]

(1) *Psychic experiences* are those in which we learn about or influence the world through means other than the conventionally recognised senses (e.g. extra-sensory perception/ESP, mind over matter).

(2) *Mystical experiences* are those in which there is a strong sense of greater connection, sometimes amounting to union, with the divine, other people, other life forms, objects, surroundings or the universe itself. Often, this is accompanied by a sense of ecstasy.

(3) *Peak experiences* are moments when people experience, more closely than usual, all that one can be. One may feel in the flow of things, self-fulfilled, engaged in optimal functioning and filled with the highest happiness. They may be triggered by art, sport, music, the natural world, tragedy or noble acts.

(4) *Out of body experiences (OBEs)* involve a sensation of being outside one's body and, in some cases, perceiving the physical body from a place outside the body.

(5) *Hauntings* are characterised by subjective visions ('ghosts') and sometimes noises in a particular location.

(6) *Poltergeist activity* is usually associated with a person rather than a place and involves phenomena, such as destruction/relocation of furniture, levitation of cutlery, knocking on doors, unusual noises.

(7) *Experiences of unusual healing* include instances of recovery, cure or enhancement of physical, psychological or spiritual well-being beyond what is usually experienced or expected on the basis of conventional medical or psychological knowledge (e.g. psychic healing or distant healing).

(8) *Encounter experiences* are those in which the person is confronted with something that is actually there but is awesome and wondrous (e.g. a glorious mountain peak) or something that is not supposed to be there (e.g. UFOs, angels, mythical beings, spirit guides).

(9) *Reincarnation/past life experiences* include the belief that the soul or spirit has been reborn into another body.

(10) *Therianthropy* is the belief that one can transform into an animal and often involves experiencing phantom limbs (feeling as though a body part is missing) or mental shifts (altered state of consciousness).

(11) *Synchronicity* is defined as a meaningful connection between an inner event (e.g. thought, vision, dream) and one or more external events occurring at the same time. For example, thinking about someone and that person then phoning you to tell you something important.

(12) *Spiritual crisis* often occurs after a spiritual experience or after intense spiritual practice (e.g. meditation, yoga) and can cause the person to question their beliefs, values and meaning system.

(13) *Alien abduction* involves memories of being taken by apparently nonhuman entities and subjected to physical and/or psychological procedures.

(14) *Near death experiences (NDEs)* typically occur to individuals close to death or in dangerous situations and often involve sensations of detachment from the body, feelings of levitation and the presence of a light.

(15) *Unusual death related experiences* include strange experiences associated with the moment of death, such as clocks stopping, mediumship, apparitions of the deceased, feeling a sense of presence and communication with the deceased.

The paranormal as an unhelpful concept in psychotherapy and counselling research

Rose Cameron

ABSTRACT

This paper, which opens with a description of what might be considered an instance of extrasensory perception in the therapeutic encounter, argues that the concepts of extrasensory perception and the paranormal are embedded in a debate in which therapists need not become involved. It argues that the discipline of parapsychology, and therefore the terms 'paranormal' and 'extrasensory perception' are embedded within a scientific narrative. In seeking to become accepted by the scientific establishment, parapsychology has entered into a debate with that establishment. This debate is of no consequence to therapeutic practice: the search for objectivity is irrelevant to understanding what happens in the therapeutic encounter. This paper suggests that the subjective basis of Phenomenology is more appropriate to psychotherapy and counselling research. It analyses the opening account and suggests that phenomenological description enables us to uncover some of the richness – and oddness – of the therapeutic encounter. The senses and the imagination are not separate faculties, but entangled in a way that enables us to make contact with the hidden or invisible aspects of the world. A phenomenological attitude of 'curiosity and disciplined naiveté' enables us to understand something of the complex, subtle and sometimes uncanny nature of communication and perception.

Das Paranormale: Ein nicht hilfreiches Konzept in der Psychotherapie- und Beratungsforschung

Der Artikel beginnt mit der Beschreibung eines Falles, der sich gleichsam als transzendente Erfahrung in der therapeutischen Arbeit charakterisieren lässt. Im Anschluss daran wird dargelegt, dass Konzepte wie das Paranormale oder übersinnlicher Erfahrungen Teil von Debatten sind, an denen Therapeuten nicht teilhaben sollten. Darüber hinaus wird erörtert, dass der Zweig der Parapsychologie, mit ihren Begriffen des 'Paranormalen' und der 'transzendenten Erfahrungen', in wissenschaftliche Diskurse eingebettet sind. Um von der wissenschaftlichen Gemeinschaft akzeptiert zu werden, suchen die Vertreter der Parapsychologie das Gespräch mit diesen – allerdings sollten sich Therapeuten nicht darauf einlassen. Die Suche nach Objektivität ist dabei irrelevant in Bezug auf die therapeutische Begegnung. Der Artikel schlägt stattdessen vor, dass das subjektive

Fundament der Phänomenologie weitaus passender für die Psychotherapie- und Beratungsforschung ist. Hierzu wird die Bedeutung eines relationalen Ereignisses näher analysiert (das man als paranormal bezeichnen könnte). Die phänomenologische Darstellung ermöglicht es uns, die Reichhaltigkeit – und Sonderbarkeit – der therapeutischen Arbeit freizulegen. Das Sinnliche und das Transzendente sind nicht zwei getrennte Bereiche, sondern in einer Weise miteinander verschränkt, die es uns ermöglicht, auch mit den versteckten oder unsichtbaren Dingen der Welt in Kontakt zu kommen. Eine phänomenologische, d.h. 'neugierige und kontrolliert naive' Haltung gibt uns die Möglichkeit, etwas von der komplexen, subtilen und manchmal auch unheimlichen Natur von Kommunikation und Wahrnehmung zu verstehen.

Lo paranormal: un concepto inútil en psicoterapia y en orientación psicológica.

Este artículo comienza con una descripción de lo que puede ser considerado como una instancia de percepción extrasensorial en el encuentro terapéutico; discute que los conceptos de percepción extrasensorial y lo paranormal están insertos en un debate en el cual los terapeutas no necesitan inmiscuirse. Se discute que la disciplina de parapsicología y por lo tanto los términos 'paranormal' y 'percepción extrasensorial' han sido incluidos en una narrativa científica para tratar de ser aceptados en este ambiente, habiendo sido la parapsicología quien ha iniciado un debate en el cual, repetimos, los psicoterapeutas no necesitan participar. La búsqueda de objetividad es irrelevante para comprender lo que ocurre en el encuentro terapéutico. El artículo sugiere que las bases subjetivas de la epistemología son más adecuadas a la investigación en psicoterapia y en orientación psicológica. Se analiza un ejemplo de un incidente relacional que pudiera ser calificado como paranormal y se sugiere que la descripción fenomenológica nos permite descubrir algo de la riqueza y de lo extraño del encuentro terapéutico. Sensibilidad e imaginación no son facultades separadas sino que están involucradas entre sí de una manera que nos permite hacer contacto con los aspectos escondidos e invisibles del mundo. Una actitud fenomenológica de 'curiosidad' e 'ingenuidad disciplinada' nos permite comprender algo de la naturaleza compleja, sutil y a veces misteriosa de la comunicación y la percepción.

Il Paranormale: un concetto non utile nella ricerca in Psicoterapia e Counselling

Questo contributo, che si apre con una descrizione di quello che potrebbe essere considerato un caso di percezione extrasensoriale nell'incontro terapeutico, sostiene che i concetti di percezione extrasensoriale e paranormale siano parte di un dibattito in cui i terapeuti non dovrebbero essere coinvolti. Si sostiene che la disciplina della parapsicologia, e quindi i termini 'paranormale' e 'percezione extrasensoriale' siano immessi entro una narrazione scientifica. Nel tentativo di farsi accettare dalla comunità scientifica, la parapsicologia ha intrapreso un dibattito con l'establishment scientifico: si tratta di un dibattito in cui i terapeuti non hanno bisogno di essere coinvolti. La ricerca di oggettività è irrilevante per comprendere ciò che accade nell'incontro terapeutico. Questo contributo suggerisce che più appropriata alla ricerca in psicoterapia e nel counselling sia la soggettività che caratterizza la fenomenologia. Si analizza il resoconto di un incidente relazionale che potrebbe essere definito paranormale e si evidenzia come la descrizione fenomenologica ci permetta di scoprire la ricchezza – e la stranezza – dell'incontro terapeutico. I sensi e l'immaginazione non sono facoltà separate, ma intrecciate in modo da permetterci di entrare in contatto con gli aspetti nascosti o invisibili del mondo. Un atteggiamento fenomenologico di 'curiosità e ingenuità disciplinate' ci permette di capire qualcosa della natura complessa, sottile e talvolta inquietante della comunicazione e della percezione

Le paranormal: un concept inutile pour la recherche en psychothérapie

Avec en ouverture une description de ce qui peut être considéré comme un cas de perception extrasensorielle dans le cadre d'une rencontre thérapeutique, cet article soutient que les concepts de perception extrasensorielle et de paranormal sont pris dans un débat auquel les thérapeutes n'ont aucunement besoin de prendre part. Il soutient que la parapsychologie, et donc les termes de 'paranormal' et de 'perception extrasensorielle', sont pris dans un discours scientifique. Dans sa recherche d'acceptation par l'establishment scientifique, la parapsychologie est entrée dans un débat avec ledit establishment : c'est un débat qui ne devrait pas concerner les thérapeutes. La recherche d'objectivité n'est pas pertinente pour comprendre ce qui se passe dans la rencontre thérapeutique. Cet article suggère que le fondement subjectif de la phénoménologie est plus approprié pour aborder la recherche en psychothérapie et counselling. L'article analyse le récit d'un incident relationnel qu'on pourrait qualifier de paranormal et suggère que la description phénoménologique nous permet de dévoiler une partie de la richesse – et de l'étrangeté – de la rencontre thérapeutique. Sens et imagination ne sont pas des aptitudes distinctes mais au contraire entremêlées, qui nous permettent d'entrer en contact avec les aspects caché et invisibles du monde. Une attitude phénoménologique 'de curiosité et de naïveté disciplinée' nous permet de comprendre quelque chose de la nature complexe, subtile et parfois étrange de la communication et de la perception.

Το παραφυσικό: Μια μη βοηθητική έννοια στην Έρευνα της Ψυχοθεραπείας και της Συμβουλευτικής

ΠΕΡΙΛΗΨΗ Το παρόν άρθρο, το οποίο ξεκινά με μια περιγραφή του τι θα μπορούσε να θεωρηθεί ως παράδειγμα της διαισθητικής αντίληψης στη θεραπευτική συνάντηση, υποστηρίζει ότι οι έννοιες της διαισθητικής αντίληψης και του παραφυσικού ενσωματώνονται σε μια συζήτηση στην οποία οι θεραπευτές δεν χρειάζεται να εμπλακούν. Υποστηρίζει ότι ο τομέας της παραψυχολογίας, και ως εκ τούτου οι όροι «παραφυσικό» και «διαισθητική αντίληψη» είναι ενσωματωμένος μέσα σε μια επιστημονική αφήγηση. Στην προσπάθειά της να γίνει δεκτή από το επιστημονικό κατεστημένο, η παραψυχολογία έχει εισέλθει σε μια συζήτηση με αυτό: είναι μια συζήτηση στην οποία οι θεραπευτές δεν χρειάζεται να εμπλακούν. Η αναζήτηση για την αντικειμενικότητα είναι άνευ σημασίας για την κατανόηση αυτού που συμβαίνει στη θεραπευτική συνάντηση. Αυτό το άρθρο δείχνει ότι η υποκειμενική βάση της Φαινομενολογίας είναι πιο κατάλληλη για την έρευνα της ψυχοθεραπείας και της συμβουλευτικής. Αναλύει μια έκθεση ενός σχεσιακού περιστατικού που θα μπορούσε να ονομαστεί παραφυσικό, και προτείνει ότι η φαινομενολογική περιγραφή παρέχει τη δυνατότητα να αποκαλύψει κάτι από τον πλούτο -και το αλλόκοτο- της θεραπευτικής συνάντησης. Η λογική και η φαντασία δεν είναι ξεχωριστές ικανότητες, αλλά εμπλεκόμενες σε έναν τρόπο που μας δίνει τη δυνατότητα να έρθουμε σε επαφή με τις κρυφές ή αόρατες πτυχές του κόσμου. Μια φαινομενολογική στάση «περιέργειας και πειθαρχημένης αφέλειας» μας επιτρέπει να καταλάβουμε κάτι από την πολύπλοκη, διακριτική και μερικές φορές παράξενη φύση της επικοινωνίας και της αντίληψης.

> It is only with such an attitude of openness and wonder that we can encounter
> the impenetrable everyday mysteries. (van Deurzen-Smith, 1997, p. 5)

Some years ago, a new client, whom I shall call Mary, was talking about her manager's response to a dilemma that had emerged in the course of her work. As she was recounting their conversation, I ... I want to say I 'saw', but perhaps 'perceived' might be more accurate ... I perceived ... something ... wiggling across the short distance between us. It was an invisible something, yet I somehow perceived it to have a form. It was rather like an elongated (and wriggly) jellybean: translucent, yet somehow also encased in a slightly opaque shell. It had a very distinct emotional quality of repeated, heart-sinking disappointment.

In trying to describe this experience, I am aware that it sounds bizarre, yet at the time it was not distractingly so. I assumed that, as the wiggly jellybean was a few inches in front of her chest, its quality of heart-sinking disappointment had something to do with Mary. That she might feel disappointed did not make sense to me in the context of what she was saying, so it was with greater tentativeness than usual that I asked if that was how she felt. She paused, rolled her eyes and compared her manager's failure to guide her in her present situation to her parent's failure to guide her in childhood. She talked with passion about feeling let down – again.

The idea that a therapist might access a client's unspoken feelings is fundamental to many schools of counselling and psychotherapy and variously theorised. However, my experience with the jellybean seems to be outwith these theories. It cannot be understood as projective identification or as embodied counter-transference as I did not experience Mary's disappointment within myself. The jellybean was most definitely 'out there', wriggling in the space between us. *I* did not feel disappointed.

Given that Mary identified with the disappointment, my experience with the jellybean *can* be conceptualised as empathy at the edge of the client's awareness (Rogers, 1966). However, the means by which I reach empathic understanding usually involve an interplay of listening to what my client says and how they say it; consciously or unconsciously noticing their non-verbal expressions; understanding their frame of reference and prior experience and attending to my own embodied experience. It does not usually involve an apparently disembodied emotion wriggling through the air.

My experience could, perhaps, be considered an example of extrasensory perception, and as such, as an aspect of the paranormal. The parapsychologist Beloff (1974) defines the paranormal as 'phenomena which in one or more respects conflict with accepted scientific opinion as to what is physically possible' (p. 1). Disembodied emotion that wriggles in space in the form of an elongated jellybean-like thing would certainly seem to be in conflict with accepted scientific opinion as to what is physically possible, as would perceiving such a thing.

My jellybean experience is just one of many anecdotes that I could relate about bizarre experiences in the therapeutic encounter. I suspect that the same could be said for many other practitioners. I know I am not the only therapist to have seen misty outlines around a client, or to have seen a client's face change into other faces as we speak – becoming very old, very young, acquiring or losing facial hair, looking like an entirely different person. Accounts of these kinds of experiences rarely appear in the literature, and on those occasions in which I have heard others talk of them, they have generally done so with an air of slightly spooked puzzlement. This special issue on the paranormal invites discussion of such experiences. Although I welcome the invitation, I will, in this paper, argue that the paranormal is not a helpful concept in discussing what happens in the therapeutic relationship.

Parapsychology

I make this argument not because I think that belief in the paranormal is stupid (Smith, Foster, & Stovin, 1998), naïve (Bainbridge, 1978; Lamont, 2006; Wuthnow, 1976) or indicative of psychosis (Thalbourne, 1994; Thalbourne & Delin, 1994; Williams & Irwin, 1991), but because the concept of the paranormal arises from, and is embedded in a tussle in which therapists simply need not become embroiled.

The term 'paranormal' – and the associated term 'extrasensory perception' – was brought into the English language by J.B Rhine of Duke University (who also coined the term 'parapsychology'). The Oxford English Dictionary (2016) hints at the concept's origins in referring to the paranormal as 'supposed psychical events and phenomena', the 'psychical' being related to 'psychic' rather than 'psychological'. The paranormal has its conceptual origins in what Collins and Pinch (1979) call 'the murky world of Spiritualism' (p. 255) – and herein lies the origin of the tussle.

Some involved in nineteenth-/early twentieth-century Spiritualism, notably Helena Blavatsky, founder of Theosophy, a school of mysticism that has deeply influenced the contemporary New Age, took an ideological stand against what Blavatsky called 'materialist science' (Washington, 1993). Others sought to establish scientific evidence for the 'steady stream of puzzling phenomena' that the British parapsychologist Beloff (1993) says 'cried out for impartial investigation' (p. 39). Beloff tells us that much of the steady stream of puzzling phenomena was 'of a physical nature' – raps on the séance table that spelt out coded messages, the playing of musical instruments by unseen hands, the movement of objects and furniture by an invisible agency, levitation of furniture, and occasionally people, the intrusion of objects into the séance room, the sudden displacement of an object from one locale to another and the materialisation, firstly of hands, but, in the 1870s, 'full form materializations, such as were ultimately to become indistinguishable from a living human being' (p. 42).

Given the prominence of such phenomena in the séance rooms of the late nineteenth-century period, it was, says Beloff, not surprising that it was physicists who were most keen to investigate what must have looked like a new force in nature. That all such phenomena lack credibility, he concludes, 'goes without saying' and he notes that, bar the odd poltergeist, there is nothing comparable in contemporary Spiritualism. Rhine introduced the term 'paranormal' in an attempt to distance the objects of his scientific investigation from the Spiritualist context in which they had emerged. He was instrumental in establishing the first experimental laboratory, at Duke University in the 1930s, and from this point in time, parapsychologists positioned themselves within academia, while non-academics have continued the tradition of psychical research, which largely consists of testing psychics and mediums. Some parapsychologists investigate intellectual, psychological and social characteristics that underlie a belief in the paranormal,[1] while others use the methods of experimental psychology to investigate the objective validity of paranormal phenomena such as telepathy.

To say that experimental parapsychology is unwelcome within academia would be something of an understatement. Collins and Pinch (1979) analyse the ways in which contemporary parapsychologists have sought to gain scientific recognition for their discipline and its findings, and 'the tactics used by orthodox scientists to deny them this stamp of legitimacy' (p. 238). Early experiments in which research subjects guess the order of a randomly ordered pack of cards while being isolated from any possible sensory channel of communication with the cards, or anyone knowing the order of the cards have, Collins and Pinch (1979) tell us, been replaced by the generation of random targets processed by complex electronic equipment which can be tested for randomness over millions of trials. This has been accompanied by an increasing sophistication in statistical analysis and experimental techniques such as 'double blind' judging of results, and the use of independent observers. 'It seems likely that the best of modern parapsychology', say Collins and Pinch (1979), 'comprises some of the most rigorously controlled and methodologically sophisticated work in the sciences' (pp. 243–244).

The tactics that Collins and Pinch (1979) identify as being used by critics of parapsychology include,

- A blank refusal to believe. Collins and Pinch quote the physicist Helmholtz as saying:

I cannot believe it. Neither the testimony of all the Fellows of the Royal Society, nor even the evidence of my own senses would lead me to believe in the transmission of thought from one person to another independently of the recognised channels of sensation. It is clearly impossible. (p. 244)

- A refusal to publish.
- Attacks on methodological precepts. Collins and Pinch (1979) illustrate what they call this 'startling' criticism by quoting the mathematician Spencer-Brown as saying that if there is statistical evidence for paranormal phenomena, then the accepted statistical method must be called into question. 'The statistical criticisms' say Collins and Pinch (1979) 'show the length to which sceptics are prepared to go, for, were their arguments to be accepted, normal scientific statistical procedures would have to be abandoned over a wide area' (p. 248).
- Unfavourable comparisons with canonical versions of scientific method, such as the need for a theoretical explanation or the repeatability of experimental results. Collins and Pinch suggest that the criticism that parapsychology lacks credible theories is out of date. One of the central *foci* of interest in parapsychology at the moment, they say, is the theoretical debate between those advancing electromagnetic theories and those advancing quantum mechanical explanations. The criticism that parapsychologists have not produced anything like a repeatable experiment is dealt with in depth in Collins (1976); Crumbaugh (1966) and Cohen (1966).
- The fraud hypothesis, an unusual suggestion to make of colleagues' work and one against which, Collins and Pinch (1979) show, there can be no defence if it is pushed to extremes.

Many of these criticisms, say Collins and Pinch (1979), would have a devastating effect if turned against parts of orthodox science. Perhaps the most telling criticism is that based on the discipline's 'murky origins'. It would, as Collins and Pinch suggest, be unusual for modern chemistry to be criticised on the grounds that chemistry's origins lie in alchemy, or the practice of surgery to be criticised because it arose from barbering. Allison (1979) agrees that opposition to Parapsychology stems from its origins, but adds that parapsychology's continued association with occult through funding and the disciple's popular appeal does not help.

Although the reality of paranormal phenomena and the validity of parapsychology are strongly contested by the scientific establishment, the discipline of parapsychology has embedded itself within a scientific narrative. Parapsychology's aim is to demystify the paranormal. Its most basic theoretical assumption is that the objectivity-seeking methods used by experimental psychology should be able to establish the existence of paranormal phenomena. Were parapsychologists to succeed in providing evidence and theories acceptable to the scientific establishment, the phenomena they explain would, of course no longer be 'phenomena which in one or more respects conflict with accepted scientific opinion as to what is physically possible', and therefore no longer paranormal (or psychic).

Parapsychology's tussle with the scientific establishment is a tussle in which we need not become entangled. Perhaps the most interesting thing about my opening anecdote is that although the jellybean did strike me as a *little* odd, I did not find it odd enough to be distracting. I immediately made sense of it as communicating something about Mary – in fact, I found the possibility that Mary was feeling disappointed more puzzling than the arrival of a jellybean wiggling through the space between us. Had I, in the moment, become interested in whether the jellybean was paranormal or scientifically explicable, I would have done so at Mary's expense (literally). The question is irrelevant. Instead, I became interested in the disappointment, and this led to a very useful piece of work.

In becoming interested in the disappointment rather than the jellybean, I was, of course, not doing anything unusual – most therapists would (I hope) have done the same. The communicative transactions that we have with clients happen within the context of the therapeutic relationship and mean something within that context. Whether the means of some of these transactions can be replicated under the rigorous experimental conditions imposed by parapsychologists is of little consequence in practice. Totton (2007) argues that several of the fundamental features of psychotherapy – communicative counter-transference, metabolising the patient's difficult feelings, projective identification, 'the energy in the room' – are essentially paranormal concepts. Therapists routinely set aside questions concerning the objective reality of what is experienced in intersubjective space because they just do not matter.

There are, of course, many who strive to position the theoretical concepts that we use firmly within a scientific narrative. Schore (2003), for instance, argues that the mechanism by which projective identification occurs lies in our unconscious ability to process the tiniest inflection of verbal and non-verbal communication. Such explanations are interesting in themselves, but what is perhaps of more interest is the way in which they are used. As the tussle between parapsychology and the scientific establishment makes clear, evidence and the theories that arise from it – and the theories that we set out to provide evidence for – are produced in a political context. Like parapsychology, psychotherapy has (largely) positioned itself within a scientific narrative – and many are currently engaged in a concerted effort to embed it even further. Objective evidence may indeed be useful in our relationship with funders, but it is the subjective experience of the therapeutic encounter that is important in our relationship with clients. The search for objective evidence (that therapy 'works', that what happens in the therapeutic encounter is 'real') leads us both towards, but also away from an understanding of what it is that we do. I am, in the rest of this paper, going to argue that it is of more value in our relationship with clients to practice a science that is grounded in the subjective.

Phenomenology

The philosopher Edmund Husserl (1859–1938) established Phenomenology as such a science. He was critical of Positivist science as, amongst other things, being compromised by the assumption that the natural world and its contents are given and do not need to be questioned (Crease, 2012). In Phenomenology, the field of investigation is the everyday world as we experience it. Thus, Phenomenologists forego the dualism of subject and object by looking at how things show themselves to us.

Examining the world as we experience it involves putting to one side the pre-understandings with which we normally filter our experience. Husserl conceived of this process of 'bracketing' or 'phenomenological reduction' as involving two elements: knowing that one is using filters, and putting them aside (Cogan, 2006). The first phenomenological reduction that Husserl proposes is that of the natural sciences. The scientific reduction reduces the field of investigation to phenomena as they are experienced, rather than as how they may be proven or measured. The second reduction, of the natural attitude, brackets taken-for-granted, everyday ideas about what is and is not real. Phenomenologists aim to let the things we experience appear in our consciousness as if for the first time (Landridge, 2007). The paradox is that in order to see naturally, we must let go of our preconceptions as to what is 'natural'. The psychological reduction aims to pre-empt explanation and to instead simply to describe what is in conscious experience. The focus of the psychological reduction is on the subjective meanings that phenomena have for us. The transcendental reduction and eidetic reduction, or intuition of essences, involve a radical standing aside from one's subjective experience and ego in order to discern the invariant characteristics and meanings of a phenomenon without which it would not be the thing itself.

Finlay (2011) tells us that the process of bracketing is sometimes wrongly understood to be an exercise in objectivity, but that rather than striving to be unbiased, distanced or detached, phenomenologists aim to be fully engaged, involved, interested in and open to what may appear. She draws a parallel with psychotherapy in that as therapists,

> we use ourselves as tools in the therapy and subtly intertwine with our clients exploring their sense of self and lived worldly experience. We accept that the only access we have to the other's unconscious and implicit meanings is through the 'between'. (p. 22)

Husserl's process of bracketing shows us, she says, how to perceive and reflect in a more complex, layered and expansive manner, turning the tables on the

traditional scientific understanding of reduction as a narrowing or abstract-
ing process. There is (unsurprisingly) a debate within phenomenology as to
whether one *can* put aside one's cultural and historical filters. Hermeneutic
Phenomenology, the branch of Phenomenology that argues that one cannot,
emphasises the inevitability of interpretation and the importance of reflexivity.
It is, I think, surprising that a methodology rooted ontologically in the subjective
and intersubjective, and which emphasises the importance of reflexivity is not
more often used in psychotherapy and counselling research.

Phenomenology values description as illuminating the complexity and richness of experience, and phenomenological description is a means by which we
might learn more about what actually happens in the therapeutic encounter.
My account of perceiving Mary's disappointment as a wriggly jellybean is an
example of this. The first three of the reductions described above are evident
(and it is the first three that are generally used in phenomenological research as
opposed to phenomenological philosophy). I put the scientific attitude aside in
that I did not, when sitting with her, think of Mary as a collection of symptoms.
Rather, I experienced being in her presence. That I also performed the reduction
of the natural attitude in putting questions of what is ordinarily considered real
to one side is clear: I saw/felt/perceived a jelly bean thingy in air, and did not find
this particularly odd. My account also illustrates the psychological reduction in
that I did not try to explain why I was seeing a jellybean wriggling through the
air – I just described what I saw/felt/perceived.

Totton (2007) calls empathy and intuition 'quietly mysterious phenomena',
and that is, what they prove to be if we approach them with a phenomenological attitude of 'curiosity and disciplined naiveté' (Giorgi, 1985; cited in Finlay,
2011). My account of working with Mary seems bizarre only because I gave a
detailed description of what I experienced. I might simply have said that I had
empathised with her, or that I had intuited her disappointment. Rich phenomenological description enables us to understand something of the complex,
subtle and sometimes uncanny nature of communication and perception. We
are, I think, all aware of taking in more than a client's words, yet research into the
experience of perception from the point of view of psychotherapy and counselling is relatively scant. 'We need', says Carl Rogers (1980) in writing about
extrasensory perception, 'to learn more about our intuitive abilities, our capacity
for sensing with the whole organism' (p. 313).

The phenomenologist, Maurice Merleau-Ponty (1945/1962) says that '(n)oth-
ing can be more difficult than to know precisely what we see' and that 'perception hides itself from itself' (p. 58). However, we can, under certain conditions,
become aware of our perceptual process. We are, for instance, generally aware of
the objects in a room rather than the way in which light falls upon them, but we
can become aware of the quality of light. The premise of the Impressionist project in European art was predicated on the idea that what we see is light falling
upon an object; Monet's haystacks are a ready example of how the same object

looks very different in different lights. While it is the case, within a reductionist scientific narrative, that what we see is light falling on an object, this explanation does not account for the interpretative nature of perception. Merleau-Ponty argues that the process of perception brings about a whole, a gestalt in which we make sense of what we see. The post-impressionist Cézanne's genius, he says in a later essay, is that:

> when the over-all composition of the picture is seen globally, perspectival distortions are no longer visible in their own right but rather contribute, as they do in natural vision, to the impression of an emerging order, of an object in the act of appearing, organizing itself before our eyes. (1948/1964, p. 14)

We do not see as a camera sees, but adjust what we see in order that it makes sense, that it looks 'right'. Dreyfus (2005) illustrates this argument by pointing out that in a 'selfie' photograph, one's nose often seems extraordinarily large because it is nearest to the lens. It is also usually the part of the face that is nearest a mirror, but one does not perceive one's nose as bizarrely large when looking in a mirror. Although I did not waste Mary's time (and money) by trying to explain the jellybean to myself, I did make meaning of it. I understood it as having something to do with Mary. Perception is an interpretative process.

A phenomenological account of perception also speaks of its embodied and synaesthetic nature. Merleau-Ponty (1945/1962) shows that perception is a bodily process rather than a mental process that happens just outside the bounds of what our minds do (Dreyfus, 2005). Merleau-Ponty's pre-conceptual and pre-linguistic account of perception has us engaging with other people via 'intercorporality', or our bodily involvement with each other, rather than working things out by thinking about them or using linguistic constructs (infectious yawning is an example of intercorporality). The body, for Merleau-Ponty, is inseparable from the world in which it is immersed and entangled: body and world are not separate. For reasons that are irrelevant to the account, Mary and I were sitting much closer together than we usually did, or as I usually sit with a client. I have always had a suspicion that my perceiving the jellybean had something to do with our physical proximity, almost as if she extended into a space around her, and that I too had extended into that space.

If I ask myself which sense I used in order to sense the disappointment conveyed by the jellybean, I would have to say that I don't know, but that I somehow sensed it with my whole body – or perhaps with an outwardly attuned sensitivity that nestles behind the flesh of my torso. And the jellybean itself? I saw that – sort of. I did not see it in quite the same way as I saw Mary, but nor was it purely a mental picture. It seemed to inhabit a space between the physical and the imaginative. Abrams (1996) tells us that that the imagination is not a separate mental faculty, but rather an attribute of the senses and is,

> the way the senses themselves have of throwing themselves beyond what is immediately given, in order to make tentative contact with the other sides of things that we do not sense directly, with the hidden or invisible aspects of the sensible. (p. 58)

Conclusion

My senses threw themselves beyond what Mary told me; they threw themselves into her psychic space. This is, in therapy at least, not in the slightest bit unusual. The concept of extrasensory perception is only necessary from within a world view that reduces perception to a camera-like mechanism, and that does not take account of the photographer. A phenomenological account of the therapeutic encounter shows that the ways in which we perceive a client are interpretive, multisensory, complex, sometimes elusive. They trouble the boundaries between body and mind. Therapists' perception happens in the context of the therapeutic relationship, and is meaningful in that context. What may or may not happen in the experimental laboratory is of little consequence.

Note

1. See the earlier references to Smith et al. (1998); Blackmore (1997); Otis and Alcock (1982) for intellectual characteristics; Thalbourne (1994); Thalbourne and Delin (1994); Williams and Irwin (1991), and to Auton, Pope, and Seeger (2003); Thalbourne (1995); Blackmore and Moore (1994); Brugger et al. (1993); Irwin (1992); Lawrence, Edwards, Barraclough, Church, and Hetherington (1995) for psychological characteristics and Wuthnow (1976); Emmons and Sobal (1981); Tobacyk, Miller, Murphy, and Mitchell (1988) and Randall (1990) for social characteristics.

References

Abrams, D. (1996). *The spell of the sensuous*. London: Vintage.

Allison, P. D. (1979). Experiemental parapsychology as a ejected science. In R. Wallis (Ed.), *On the margins of science: The social construction of rejected knowledge* (pp. 271–291). Keele: Sociological Review Monograph 27.

Auton, H., Pope, J., & Seeger, G. (2003). It isn't that strange: Paranormal belief and personality traits. *Social Behavior and Personality: An International Journal, 31*, 711–719.

Bainbridge, W. S. (1978). Chariots of the gullible. *Skeptical Inquirer, 3*, 33–48.

Beloff, J. (1974). *New directions in parapsychology*. London: Elek.

Beloff, J. (1993). *Parapsychology: A concise history*. London: Athlone Press.

Blackmore, S. (1997). Probability misjudgment and belief in the paranormal: A newspaper survey. *British Journal of Psychology, 88*, 683–689.

Blackmore, S., & Moore, R. (1994). Seeing things: Visual recognition and belief in the paranormal. *European Journal of Parapsychology, 88*, 683–689.

Brugger, P., Regard, M., Landis, T., Cook, N., Krebs, D., & Niederberger, J. (1993). 'Meaningful' patterns in visual noise: Effects of lateral stimulation and the observer's belief in ESP. *Psychopathology, 26*, 261–265.

Cogan, J. (2006). The phenomenological reduction. *Internet Encyclopaedia of Philosophy*. Retrieved from http://www.iep.utm.edu/phen-red/

Cohen, D. (1966, May 9). E.S.P. science or delusion? *The Nation*, p. 550–553.

Collins, H. M. (1976). *Upon the replication of scientific findings: A discussion illuminated by the experiences of researchers into parapsychology.* Paper read at the S.S.S.S., I.S.A. Conference, Cornell University, Ithaca, NY.

Collins, H. M., & Pinch, T. J. (1979). The construction of the paranormal: Nothing unscientific is happening. In R. Wallis (Ed.), *On the margins of science: The social construction of rejected knowledge* (pp. 243–244). Keele: Sociological Review Monograph 27.

Crease, R. P. (2012). Phenomenology and natural science. *Encyclopaedia of Philosophy*. Retrieved from http://www.iep.utm.edu/phenomsc/

Crumbaugh, J. C. (1966). A scientific critique of parapsychology. *International Journal of Neuropsychiatry, 2*, 539–555.

Dreyfus, H. (2005). *Philosophy 188: Merleau-Ponty's phenomenology of perception* [Online]. Retrieved June 7, 2014, from http://ist-socrates.berkeley.edu/~hdreyfus/188_s05/html/Lectures.html

Emmons, C. F., & Sobal, J. (1981). Paranormal beliefs: Testing the marginality hypothesis. *Sociological Focus, 14*, 49–56.

Finlay, L. (2011). *Phenomenology for therapists* (1st ed.). London: John Wiley.

Giorgi, A. (Ed.). (1985). *Phenomenological and psychological research*. Pittsburgh, PA: Duquesne University Press.

Irwin, H. J. (1992). Origins and functions of paranormal belief: The role of childhood trauma and interpersonal control. *Journal of the American Society for Psychical Research, 86*, 199–208.

Lamont, P. (2006). Critically thinking about paranormal belief. In S. Della Sala (Ed.), *Tall tales: Popular myths about the mind and brain* (pp. 23–35). Oxford: Oxford University Press.

Landridge, D. (2007). *Phenomenological psychology*. Harlow: Pearson.

Lawrence, T. R., Edwards, C., Barraclough, N., Church, S., & Hetherington, F. (1995). Modelling childhood causes of paranormal belief and experience: Childhood trauma and childhood fantasy. *Personality and Individual Differences, 19*, 209–215.

Merleau-Ponty, M. ([1945] published in English 1962). *Phenomenology of perception*. (C. Smith, Trans.). London: Routledge and Kegan Paul.

Merleau-Ponty, M. ([1948] published in English 1964). *Sense and non-sense*. Evanston, IL: Northwestern University Press.

Otis, L. P., & Alcock, J. (1982). Factors affecting extraordinary belief. *The Journal of Social Psychology, 118*, 77–85.

Oxford English Dictionary. (2016). Retrieved March 1, 2016, from http://www.oed.com

Randall, T. M. (1990). Belief in the paranormal declines: 1977–1987. *Psychological Reports, 66*, 1347–1351.

Rogers, C. R. (1966). Client-centred therapy. In S. Arieti (Ed.), *American handbook of psychiatry* (pp. 183–200). New York, NY: Basic Books.

Rogers, C. R. (1980). *A way of being*. Boston, MA: Houghton Mifflin.

Schore, A. (2003). *Affect regulation and the repair of the self*. London: Norton.

Smith, M. D., Foster, C. L., & Stovin, G. (1998). Intelligence and paranormal belief: Examining the role of context. *Journal of Parapsychology, 62*, 65–77.

Thalbourne, M. A. (1994). Belief in the paranormal and its relationship to schizophrenia-relevant measures: A confirmatory study. *British Journal of Clinical Psychology, 33,* 78–80.

Thalbourne, M. A. (1995). Further studies of the measurement and correlates of belief in the paranormal. *Journal of the American Society for Psychical Research, 89,* 233–247.

Thalbourne, M. A., & Delin, P. S. (1994). A common thread underlying belief in the paranormal, creative personality, mystical experience and psychopathology. *Journal of Parapsychology, 58,* 3–38.

Tobacyk, J., Miller, M., Murphy, P., & Mitchell, T. (1988). Comparisons of paranormal beliefs of black and white university students from the southern United States. *Psychological Reports, 63,* 492–494.

Totton, N. (2007). Funny you should say that: Paranormality, at the margins and the centre of psychotherapy. *European Journal of Psychotherapy & Counselling, 9,* 389–401.

van Deurzen-Smith, E. (1997). *Everyday mysteries: Existential dimensions of psychotherapy.* London: Routledge.

Washington, P. (1993). *Madam Blavatsky's Baboon: A history of the mystics, mediums and misfits who brought spiritualism to America.* New York, NY: Schocken.

Williams, L. M., & Irwin, H. J. (1991). A study of paranormal belief, magical ideation as an index of schizotypy and cognitive style. *Personality and Individual Differences, 12,* 1339–1348.

Wuthnow, R. (1976). Astrology and marginality. *Journal for the Scientific Study of Religion, 15,* 157–168.

Phantom narratives and the uncanny in cultural life: psychic presences and their shadows

Samuel Kimbles

ABSTRACT

In this paper the author explores the emotional factors that are activated at the level of the cultural unconscious, that produce experiences of the uncanny that are expressed through Phantom Narratives. Phantom Narratives as a hybridized term is the author's way of linking personal and social activity of unconscious story formation through psychic presences (images). Phantom Narratives are expressions of the unconscious at the level of the group that shows the psyche's way of narrating its relationship to the group, through the expressions of cultural, social, and political issues. The uncanny, at the level of the social, is seen as those disturbances of feelings that alienate us from the familiar social world of others. What is uncanny about Phantom Narratives is how group emotional dynamics are represented as psychic presences. Making use of the author's own subjectivity (i.e. psychoanalytic literary genre) he uses an approach from analytic psychology (Jungian) called amplification, which allows for the elaboration of symbolic processes, to create a meaningful (semantic) context for exploration.

Phantomnarrative und das Außergewöhnliche des Kulturlebens: Übersinnliche Erscheinungen und ihre Schatten

In diesem Artikel spürt der Autor emotionalen Faktoren nach, die auf der Ebene des kulturell Unbewussten aktiviert werden. Sie produzieren, so die These, ein Unbehagen, das über sogenannte Phantomnarrative transportiert wird. Mit dem Begriff Phantomnarrativ wird versucht, eine Verbindung zwischen personalen und gesellschaftlichen Modi der unbewussten Organisation der Geschichte durch übersinnliche Erscheinungen herzustellen. Phantomnarrative sind ein Ausdruck des Unbewussten auf Gruppenebene; sie verdeutlichen, wie das Übersinnliche über Narrationen, die kulturelle, soziale und politische Aspekte betreffen, mit der Gruppe im Zusammenhang stehen. Das Unheimliche, auf Ebene der Gesellschaft lässt sich als Störung von Gefühlen begreiflich machen, die uns von unserer sonst gewohnten Umwelt entfremden. Was Phantomnarrative so außergewöhnlich macht, ist die Frage, wie emotionale Dynamiken einer Gruppe als übersinnliche Erscheinungen repräsentiert werden.

Narrativas fantasmaticas y lo misterioso / oculto en la vida cultural: presencias psíquicas y sus sombras

En este artículo el autor explora los factores emocionales que se activan a nivel del inconsciente cultural y que producen experiencias de lo extraño, las cuales se expresan a través de narrativas fantasmáticas. Narrativas fantasmáticas como un término híbrido es la manera en que el autor conecta la actividad personal y social de la formación de historias inconscientes a través de presencias psíquicas (imágenes). Las narrativas fantasmáticas son expresiones del inconsciente a nivel del grupo que muestran la manera en que la mente narra su relación con éste, a través de expresiones de aspectos culturales, sociales y políticos. Lo extraño/oculto a nivel de lo social es visto como esos trastornos del sentimiento que nos alienan del mundo social familiar de otros. Lo misterioso en las narrativas fantasmáticas es cómo las dinámicas emocionales del grupo se representan como presencias psíquicas.

Narrazioni fantasmatiche e il perturbante nella vita culturale: presenze psichiche e le loro ombre

In questo lavoro l'autore esplora i fattori emotivi che si attivano a livello dell'inconscio culturale che producono esperienze del perturbante e che si esprimono attraverso Narrazioni Fantasmatiche. Questo termine ibrido è usato dall'autore per collegare l'attività individuale e sociale relative alla storia della formazione dell'inconscio attraverso presenze psichiche (immagini). Le narrazioni fantasmatiche sono espressioni dell'inconscio a livello di gruppo che palesa il modo della psiche di raccontare la sua relazione con il gruppo, attraverso l'estrinsecazione di questioni culturali, sociali e politiche. Il perturbante, a livello del sociale, è visto come impedimento affettivo che ci allontana dal mondo sociale familiare degli altri. Ciò che è inquietante delle narrazioni fantasmatiche è come le dinamiche emotive di gruppo siano rappresentate come presenze psichiche.

Récits-fantômes et Etrangeté dans la vie culturelle : les présences psychiques et leurs ombres

Dans cet article, l'auteur explore les facteurs émotionnels qui sont activés au niveau de l'inconscient culturel et qui produisent des expériences d'étrangeté s'exprimant au travers de récits-fantômes. Le terme de récits-fantômes est un terme hybride permettant à l'auteur de lier l'activité personnelle et l'activité sociale de construction d'histoires inconscientes à travers les présences psychiques (images). Les récits-fantômes sont des expressions de l'inconscient groupal montrant la manière dont la psyché raconte sa relation au groupe à travers l'expression de problèmes culturels, sociaux et politiques. L'étrangeté, au niveau social, est perçue comme étant ces émotions perturbées qui nous coupent du monde social familier d'autrui. Ce qui est étrange avec les récits-fantômes ce sont comment les dynamiques émotionnelles du groupe sont représentées en tant que présences psychiques.

Οι Αφηγήσεις Φάντασμα και το Μυστηριώδες στην Πολιτιστική ζωή: Ψυχικές παρουσίες οι σκιές τους

Στο άρθρο αυτό ο συγγραφέας διερευνά τους συναισθηματικούς παράγοντες που ενεργοποιούνται στο επίπεδο του πολιτιστικού ασυνείδητου, οι οποίοι παράγουν εμπειρίες του ανοίκειου που εκφράζονται μέσα από τις Αφηγήσεις Φάντασμα. Οι εν λόγω αφηγήσεις ως υβριδικός όρος αφορούν τον τρόπο του συγγραφέα να συνδέει την προσωπική και κοινωνική δραστηριότητα του ασυνειδήτου σχηματισμού της ιστορίας μέσα από ψυχικές παρουσίες (εικόνες). Οι αφηγήσεις φάντασμα είναι εκφράσεις του ασυνειδήτου στο επίπεδο της ομάδας που δείχνει τον τρόπο της ψυχής να αφηγείται τη σχέση της με την ομάδα, μέσα από τις εκφράσεις των πολιτιστικών, κοινωνικών και πολιτικών ζητημάτων. Το μυστηριώδες, στο κοινωνικό επίπεδο κατανοείται ως εκείνες οι διαταραχές των συναισθημάτων που μας αποξενώνουν από τον οικείο κοινωνικό κόσμο των άλλων. Το μυστηριώδες για τις αφηγήσεις φάντασμα είναι πώς η συναισθηματική δυναμική της ομάδας αναπαρίσταται ως ψυχική παρουσία.

There is another world,

But it is in this one.

Paul Éluard

In this paper I focus on the emotional factors that are activated at the level of the cultural unconscious, producing experiences of the uncanny through what can be called Phantom Narratives, an expression of the unconscious at the level of the group appearing as individual, social and cultural dynamics. The concept of the cultural unconscious was introduced to Analytical Psychology by Joseph Henderson (1990) who defined it as 'an area of historical memory that lies between the collective unconscious and the manifest patterns of the culture' (p. 103). It may include these modalities – both consciously and unconsciously – but it derives some kind of uncanny identity arising from the archetypes of the collective unconscious, which, just as they assist in the formation of myth and ritual, also promote the process of accultured development in individuals (p. 190).

Additionally, I will apply Jung's concept of complexes to cultural processes that appear as what I have called Cultural Complexes. Complexes are naturally occurring elements in human beings that structure the individual responses to biological gives such as the body, aging, and death, and to interpersonal relations within family, tribal and broader communal systems. These naturally occurring elements are organized through affective dynamics that are often unconscious. They are the psyche's way of narrating its relationship to the group. Hence, basic cultural issues of invisibility, namelessness, marginalization, powerlessness, and rootlessness are existential issues facing all of us. When these issues are linked up with losses, racism, gender, and ethnicity, the psychology of differences comes into play along with power dynamics, as group survival seems to be at stake. Cultural Complexes are expressions of unconscious dynamics in group life serving the need to belong and have an identity by linking group expectations with personal experiences. These complex dynamics tend to function as an emotional background, but assume a certain importance and influence nonetheless as they express emotional valences for the group and the individual Kimbles, 2014; Singer & Kimbles, 2004).

Thus an understanding of Cultural Complexes allows us to understand our emotions, beliefs, and images that operate at the level of the group that contribute to the organization of group phenomena.

I see Cultural Complexes as the bones (structures) of cultural processes and Phantom Narrative as the flesh (lived experiences) of cultural experiences. In this respect, Jung puts forth a nonrational life force as the center of the human psyche:

> If we look back into the past history of mankind, we find among many other religious convictions, a universal belief in the existence of phantoms or ethereal beings who dwell in the neighborhood off men and who exercise an invisible yet powerful influence upon them. (Jung, 1981, para. 570)

The uncanny

Freud says in the opening of his paper on the Uncanny,

> Only rarely does the psychoanalyst feel impelled to engage in 'aesthetic investigations' (Freud, 1919, p.123). Later, Freud acknowledges that the term belongs to the realm of the frightening, of what evokes fear and dread … but presumes an 'affective nucleus' which justifies the use of a special conceptual term.

I see in Freud's use of the term 'affective nucleus' both a phantom echo of Jung's theory of complexes and recognition of the transpersonal emotional core of many Cultural Complexes. Freud based his analysis of the uncanny on E.T.A. Hoffman's text, *Der Sandman*, which led him to explore a number of etymological features of the term *unheimlich*, ostensibly the opposite of Heimlich – a transition from the familiar to the unfamiliar, and yet fully retaining its connection to what in the cultural life of a family one has once more consciously known.

Unheimlich (unfamiliar) though associated with the self, and known to the self yet supposed to remain hidden from the self, but has become apparent, has become visible to the self. "The unhelmlich, though unfamiliar, comes bundled with references to the self (Sadeq Rahimi, 2013, p. 459).

As for Freud's conclusion about the uncanny he says: 'we have to admit that none of this helps us to understand the extraordinarily strong feelings of something uncanny that pervades that conception' (Freud, 1919, p. 236). He concludes the origin of the uncanny as castration and the return of the repressed – the uncanny tropes are a group of phenomena 'in which the 'frightening element can be shown to be something repressed which returns' (Freud, 1919, p. 241).

The concept of the uncanny has moved far beyond Freud's understanding of it as representing the continued presence of animism, omnipotence of thought based on it, and repressed infantile complexes. It is used as a key concept to grasp the experience of political and social alienation resulting from uprootedness, disturbing unhomeliness (not just refugees and immigrants). It is under the aforementioned circumstances that the familiar become uncanny and frightening? We saw an example of this in 2001, when in the aftermath of 9/11, the fear of invasion and attack led to widespread political fear in America and generated a 'War on Terror,' conspiracy theories, fear of weapons of mass destruction, and the need for more control and repression at the expense of civil liberties. Cultural changes whether expressed through sudden political responses or long-standing historical traumas, i.e. slavery, can produce in our individual psyches disturbing feelings that alienate us from the familiar social world of others, both familiar and unfamiliar.

Later literature on the uncanny

The literature used to speak about the uncanny is replete with images that range from *doppelgangers*, alter egos, and splits to ghosts, unsettling doubling, madness, and invasive phantoms. Though Freud's interpreted the uncanny on the personal level as due to castration anxiety and infantile complexes similarly rooted in the force of early developmental issues, others have expanded its definition:

For instance, Rahimi writes:

It is also useful to consider the place of mirrors and the visual in the historical trajectory of the modern conceptions of human selfhood. This role is worth attention for two reasons: the triangular relationship between the visual the ego and the uncanny, and the social and historical embededness of the experience of subjectivity. (p. 455)

I extend the meaning of the uncanny to social and cultural processes *operating at the level of the cultural unconscious*. Gordon's (1997) reframing the uncanny in social terms is consistent with my view of the uncanny:

The social is ultimately what the uncanny is about; being haunted in the world of common reality. To be haunted is not a contest between animism and a discrediting reality test, or a contest between the unconscious and the conscious faculties. It is an enchanted encounter in a disenchanted world between familiarity and estrangement. (pp. 54–55)

To my mind, Gordon's use of haunting is quite cognate with Freud's notion of the uncanny. The recognition that a social phenomenon is involved moves repression through stages of a culture's troubled past, from suppression of 'alternative histories', to oppressed peoples' generation of new stories, and finally (and more bleakly) to 'alienation as an economic, political, psychological and existential condition'. (Masschelein, 2011, p. 136)

Phantoms and their narratives

I have recently introduced the concept of 'phantom narratives' as a hybridized term linking personal and social realms of unconscious story formation, expressing the background ambiguity of subject/object, individual/group, politics/ sociology, and personal biography and cultural history, conscious and unconscious, held together in an affective field. This affective field, I will argue, has a narrative structure that operates at the level of the cultural unconscious, and is along with particular images at the very heart of Cultural Complexes, drawing unconscious attention to unprocessed cultural history. Phantoms as images are representations at the core of these complexes, and their narratives give the complexes their dynamic agency.

Looked at from within the context of the cultural unconscious, Cultural Complexes, Phantom Narratives and the Uncanny I feel are expressions of disruptions in the unconscious at the group or cultural level of the psyche into the world of both the individual and social and/or cultural reality affecting. These disruptions affect roles, ideologies, and societal structures, while disturbing our subjective orientation – the order of things. Parallel disruptions occur at every level of psychological and sociological functioning.

In a recent movie *Phoenix* (2015), directed by Christian Petzold, we get a representation of a weaving together of the personal life of a post-concentration camp woman within the context of post World War II, Nazi destruction. As the movie opens we see a disfigured, bandage-faced woman (Nelly) who is returning to Berlin for reconstructive surgery. She wants to have her original face back even though it has been damaged and disfigured during her concentration camp ordeal, she says, 'I want to look exactly like I used to.' She is a traumatized and shattered woman who also returns to track down her husband, who may have betrayed her Jewish background to the Nazis. He was released and she was placed in a concentration camp.

She returns to the Phoenix café where she and her husband previously performed with her husband – he as the pianist and she as a singer. The husband fails to recognize Nelly, but finally wants her instead, 'I want you to play my wife' so that he can collect her unclaimed money. Nelly cooperates with his scheme as a way to get back her identity and to be recognized by her husband as some kind of partner again, especially since he is willing to share with her the fortune that he imagines to be that of a now dead woman. It was not until the end of the film that Johnny the husband, is shocked into trying to make sense of the inescapable fact that this woman, his wife, has returned from the dead, at least as her spirit, even though no one has allowed her to be herself. She has, in effect, become the phantom of her own culturally repressed past.

Looked at from the point of view of Phantoms and Narratives, the pair has lost everything, including the ability each to grant an authentic identity to the other. The reconstructive wish for a return to a previous identity so that life can be resumed as it always was (Nelly) or started anew (Johnny), is played out against the historical weight of a narrative of catastrophic destruction (lost of everything). Thus the film offers a vivid picture of the living out of a world that has all the features of the uncanny, particularly the doubling of identity, the confusion between being alive and the living dead-like existence that characterizes such extreme dislocation – the clear line of distinction is lost. The breakdown of the denial that Nelly and Johnny share, and the vague recognition of someone previously known, but who is now a stranger, constitute the denouement – a moment that is uncanny.

Masschelein (2011) in her book, The unconcept gives a description of the uncanny that is close to mine:

'The uncanny is a key concept to grasp the experience of aesthetic estrangement, political and social alienation resulting

In a deeply rooted, disturbing of unhomilness that characterizes human existence in the world but tempered by a mild, surrealistic undertones and the guise of familiarity' (2011, p. 147).

In a similar way to Masschelein, I feel that the Phantom Narrative is a basic concept that allows an imaginative way to articulate the experience of the uncanny as it manifests itself in individual and group history within the context of cultural dynamics.

Phantom narratives

Phantom Narratives are the operation of the unconscious at the group level, narrating themselves in the midst of Cultural Complexes as psychic presences of great fascination and uncanny power, What is 'uncanny' in the Phantom Narratives grows out of an affective field 'with deep and buried contents' (Chomsky, 1968) ideas of deep structures in language.

Grostein's understanding of 'psychic presences' helps to amplify the term Phantom, first introduced by Abraham and Torok (1994) though without the notion of narrative that Grotstein manages to imply:

My term psychic presences is meant to convey the experience of intrapsychic preternatural entities, which present as images or phantoms and which we, in turn, reify as real. These images of phantoms undergo a transfiguration of transmogrifications as we progress ... they evolve into symbolic images that designate the 'presence of the absence' of the object-person, that is, the presence of the legacy of the experience with the object in its absence. (Grotstein, 2000, p. xix)

By linking 'psychic presences' and 'phantoms' with a notion of their 'narratives', I propose a way of opening up an imaginative space for reflecting on the changes and impacts that our current historical situation with its 'too muchness' and disorientation brings to us as context and content for adaptation and engagement.

Phantom Narratives encode the representations of psychic presences in dynamic stories that quite literally narrate the individual's relationship to the group and group life on the one hand and the accompanying context that gives each phantomatic figure its meaning (the 'phantom narrative' is the intergenerational story placed in the context of its central image). Here, I would like to elaborate my understanding of the relationship between a Phantom Narrative and the Uncanny with a personal example, a dream I had a number of years ago when in advanced candidacy of Jungian analytical training.

> I am called to be a consultant at a meeting of three staff psychologists at a prison. Present at the meeting are three Afro-American men, all psychologists working in the prison system. The three men I identify as a colleague from graduate school, the first president of the American Black Psychologists Association, and a man who was a combination of my father and Clarence Thomas (Associate Justice of the Supreme Court). I am being asked to consult around a problem the group is grappling with which is that though mental health services have been made available and given to the black community and prisoners, the rate of young black men imprisonment remains extremely high. The psychologists have no useful explanation for this situation. They think that as an analytical psychologist I may have something to offer from an archetypal psychology point of view.

Let me give some of my conscious experience with these three men. One was trained in Humanistic Psychology and at the time of my dream was a professor at a local university. The second man had been connected with the creation of the Association of Black Psychologists formed 'in recognition of the diverse historical experiences and cultural expressions within and between peoples of African ancestry …' (Home page, www.abpsi.org, 2015). The third was a combination of my father and Clarence Thomas, a member of the US Supreme Court known for his relatively conservative views. Paradoxically, Thomas as a black justice replaced Thurgood Marshall, an active liberal attorney best known for his argument before the Supreme Court that the separate but equal doctrine was unconstitutional. Later, Marshall was appointed an Associative Justice to the Supreme Court, the first African-American to hold that position. My father, though conservative around racial matters like Thomas, emphasized and mirrored, like Marshall, the importance and role of racial pride.

My dream presents a complicated sub-group of African-American men, all psychologists, who represent a range of attitudes toward racial mental health, but they felt something was missing in their approach, for nothing they came up with could help stem the tide of the continued incarceration of young African-American men. They needed to find out from me what an archetypal attitude could add to their work. All three men focused on aspects of structural violence as manifested in economic disparity in opportunity, social and political power/

privileges differences and the effects of these disparities on mental health issues and how these show up as problems of crime.

Though I had my dream two decades ago, the facts of African-American males being incarcerated has earned America the term Mass Incarceration (see, Alexander, 2010; Cox, 2015).

The statistics referred to in an article by Robynn Cox cited (2015, p. 5) by Coates (2015) reflecting mass incarceration are staggering. The United States has the highest incarceration rate in the world; though it has 5% of the world population, it houses about 25% of the world prisoners. It incarcerates black males 20–50 times longer than the white prisoner convicted of the same drug crime.

Two and a third million men are incarcerated – about half for drug crimes. Seventy percent of men imprisoned are black and Hispanic. There are 7 million Americans, males and females, either in prison, parole, and probation mostly for selling drugs.

Professor Cox (2015), wrote in her article: 'Mass Incarceration and the Struggle for Civil Rights' that

> it is clear that crime and punishment are multidimensional problems that stem from racial prejudice justified by age-old perceptions and beliefs about African American … Public policy, criminal justice actors, society and the media, and criminal behavior have all played roles in creating what sociologist Loie Wacquant calls the hyperincarceration of black men. (P.2)

And later in the same article she says,

> failure to address the legacy of racism passed down by our forefathers and it ties to economic oppression will only result in the continued reinvention of Jim Crow … from this point of view as an extension of chattel slavery i.e. turning the Other into an object to be owned. (Cox, 2015, p. 3)

> Though quite disturbing, the abovementioned conclusions by Cox appeared to have continued the approach of the psychologists in my dream that occurred two decades ago. She does add the intergenerational transmission of unconscious racism (Cultural Complexes). As my own dream was a generation ago, I find it sad that the same dynamics that troubled my African–American psychologist colleagues continue to this present day.

Uncanny and phantom narratives

Though some psychologists and sociologists have adopted a psycho-social approach to the problems addressed in my dream, thinking now about my dream through the lens of Phantom Narratives allows me to look at a psycho-emotional-archetypal approach to the complicated intersecting of individual, cultural, and historical dynamics from the point of view of the activity of the unconscious at the level of the group, as expressed by Cultural Complexes.

Though we are likely to focus on scapegoating and splitting as operating in inter-group relating, the processes fears, fantasies, feeling that give rise to the need for these emotional processes are rarely explored. From the point of view of Phantom Narratives, group experiences of cultural processes are manifested in figures and images that structure both intra psychic and inter-subjective aspects of experiencing that bring into play cultural history, social context, beliefs, and values that affectively shape group and individual responses to these cultural and social issues.

As an imagined consultation, through my dream, this paper is an expression of another of many actual and symbolic consultations I have made in response to my dream putting to me the question of what has archetypal psychology to offer to this large social and cultural problems of race relations as it manifests in the problem of mass incarceration of young African-American men in the United States.

By bringing together some of my thoughts on what I call Phantom Narratives and Freud's ideas around the uncanny as these relate to cultural, social, and political issues I hope to open up an imaginative space for the role of affect and images to be encountered as expressions of the dynamics of those aspects of the unconscious that link psyche and culture.

Although, I have focused on African-American men, the same dynamics (scapegoating, denial of group and individual shadow, splitting, etc.) that we find in their mass incarceration are easily identifiable within other cultural groups struggling to achieve a successful relation to American identity after an early cultural history elsewhere (viz, the large group of young underemployed Latino men).

The image of the phantom haunts narratives that relate individuals to the group and the group to the individual, opening up an encounter with the uncanny at the level of the cultural unconscious.

The Phantom narrative shows what is undigested but still important in the past of a culture, and how significant, and emotionally alive it continues to be both for the individual and the group that share this past. Cultural Complexes organize such narratives, but their central phantomatic images give a specifi- cally uncanny thrust to them. I propose that Phantom Narratives constitute the unconsciousness, (at the level of the group) way of expressing in symbolic form what it is doing with the experience of social and political alienation. Bollas's term, the 'unthought known' (Bollas, 1987), aptly expresses the implicit stories that organize inter and intra-group relating.

The cultural unconscious is structured by units of experience (Cultural Complexes) that where Individual, group and societal processes, affectively come together in a tangled web of cultural, psyche and group processes that are lived out subjectively and intersubjectively.

Phantom narratives are structures of images, behaviors, and rituals that give notice to the 'social nature of the subjective life' of the group and the individ- ual relationship to the group through the various social and ritual forms (see Gordon, 2008). It is one way to understand the expression at the unconscious level of the group. The organization of group processes as Cultural Complexes refuses to accept our understanding of history as a simple linearity, opening up a space between received history and alternative narratives. The Phantom fills that space with a dynamic image of a past that refuses to accept a future that does not include it. This is how, and why, it is so uncanny.

Groups that have been marginalized and traumatized through social oppression and disenfranchisement such that there is a history of broken continuity, and group fragmentation, give birth both to Phantom Narratives and lives that are profoundly influenced by the uncanny.

The activation of Phantom Narratives as 'Phantomatic Complexes' operates in what Turner (1966) has defined as a liminal space, which we might here speak of as a place between accepted cultural narratives. Phantom Narratives refer to the affectively organized units of experience-patterns that organize the experiencing of the other when the other has been denied a place in narratives endorsed by the culture's conscious establishment. Phantom Narratives like cultural complexes are 'repetitive, resisting consciousness and collecting experiences that confirms their historical point of view' (Kimbles, 2000, 2014; Singer & Kimbles, 2004). They are traumatic images that have not been forgotten that encode, in the force of their uncanniness, only partly repressed 'historical group experiences that have taken root in the cultural unconscious of the group' (p. 7) (see Singer & Kimbles, 2004). As we have seen, they gather life and narrative force there.

Summary conclusions

Putting together Phantom Narratives and Cultural Complexes creates another hybrid term, 'Phantomatic Complexes'. This allows themes of presence and absence, visibility and invisibility, life and death to be seen as manifestation of themes related to cultural history and trauma (inheritance and memories from past generations) to both find a voice and an imaginal expression, i.e. Hiroshima, World War II and Japan's defeat, the holocaust in Germany, Slavery in America, genocide around the world and most recently the Tsunami in Fukishima. All this makes for a haunting i.e. the work of processing and dealing with these tragedies as they manifest at the unconscious level (through Phantomatic Complexes). Phantomatic Complexes are major expressions in modern cultural life of unprocessed traumatic history.

As symbolic processes, Phantomatic Complexes, I suggest, emerge from a variety of actual and symbolic Social Deaths (Patterson, 1982). As symbolic processes emerge from a variety of actual and symbolic social deaths that emerge out of the processes of social negation. The prototype of every other social negation is slavery. People are uprooted, deracinated, placed in a world of master (dominated relationship) 'a world of non-being' – history is broken, culture holding is fragmented and historical alternatives are rendered mute (Patterson, 1982). Phantom Narratives as representations of Cultural Complexes are organized around psychic figures and images that animate and connect the individual psyche to the group, its cultural history and heritage, functioning at the cultural level of the unconscious, creating by intergenerational transmission, certain tasks for the individual, group and community future generations to perform. An unresolved historical event or situation emerge from repression – a type of haunting ensues. The figures appearing in cultural complexes are phantoms and are often experienced spectrally as strange and uncanny. They are organized as phantom narratives (implicit structures) and expressed though ideologies, cultural attitudes, rituals, and moral codes.

In the clinical situation when cultural reality is minimized or disconnected from life experiences the individual experiences alienation and invisibility is made manifest in the clinical situation. From this point of view at the clinical level, transference and countertransference, enactments in analysis, Phantomatic Complexes always influence interpretations. If the analytic relationship, with its historic past its cultural trauma and potential for healing the patient's cultural heritage, and its potential for community healing, create a rich phantomatic field for exploration.

I am not, however, postulating something that we cannot feel or find in our conscious emotional repertoire. I find it uncanny, for instance, that given the relentless repetition of the Phantomatic Narrative of an obvious form of loss of freedom, and all the associated Cultural Complexes that we find in the mass incarceration of young men of color, we have managed to perpetuate a former generation's blindness to the repetition of slave history into a supposedly more enlightened time, and that we refuse to accept slavery's ongoing presence in our everyday life. We choose not to see beyond the conscious, rational Crime and Punishment narrative, and so we do not see its Phantomatic roots in slavery. To follow Freud's understanding of the uncanny to its relations to the frightening and the horrific, from *heimlich*, 'homely', that which is kept out of sight to *unnhelmlich*, the 'disturbing' expresses the movement from familiarity to strangeness (Gordon, 2008, p. 1007) through the labyrinth of cultural and institutional memory. Freud (1919) resolves the relationship between these two processes by bringing in the theory of repression: 'the uncanny is in reality nothing new, or alien, but something which is familiar and old-established in the mind and which has become alienated from it only through the return of repression' (p. 399). What does the large population of black and Latino prisoners signify? Are the non-persons, our newly initiated shadow population, rapidly becoming cultural phantoms, connecting us to the tortured, unworked through history of slavery, and its shadow of racism as a radical restriction of freedom? Though there is a feeling of having been here before, this is not simply a return under the guise of racism, but the presence in plain sight of the persons made invisible and the invisible made visible.

The repressed returns, as Freud knew, through a haunting sense that we have been here before. In Toni Morrison's Beloved (1987), the invisible returns, fed by the insatiable longing for love represented by the ghost of the murdered child 'haunted by the insatiable longing for love' (Martinez, 2009). The refusal of contemporary middle-class American culture to acknowledge its complicity with the denial and recognition of the need of the people of color is producing such phantoms today. In their narratives we can still find black people whose needs, expressed through variety of behaviors the injured feelings related to negative cultural attitudes toward them, have become intergenerational phantoms. Their narratives contribute in a major way to the obscene continuation of the mass incarceration – a story that challenges cultural blindness as much as it is caused by it.

These ghosts bring demands for recognition and reparation. These are the phantom transmissions of an earlier generation's traumatic Complexes to the contemporary American black experience.

The current outcry regarding the use of body cameras with police officers to reduce violence by allowing others to be an audience, to 'Black Lives Matter', to putting up barriers, to Hispanics immigration, to Muslim hatred, we are familiar with but feel surprised with their reoccurrence. Though benefits may eventually result from the use of body cameras by police officers, it is interesting to see how many of the recent killings of young black men have been caught on cameras and how often the interpretations by officers and public are seen through entirely different eyes. It truly is a problem of complex activated perception. It is impossible to see if the eyes (perceptions) through which we see are not reflected on. I once saw a prominently placed sign on a large semi-truck calling attention to nearby drivers behind it that 'IF YOU DON'T SEE MY MIRRORS I CAN'T SEE YOU.'

There is no end to what I could summon in my own mirrors, but I would like to close with a poetic and weighty quote from Jung (1934/1954), in referring to the opening words of the Dedication in *Faust*, says:

> 'Once more you hover near me, forms and faces' – are more than just an aesthetic flourish. Like the concretism of the devil, they are an admission of the objectivity of psychic experience, a whispered avowal that this was what actually happened, not because of subjective wishes, or fears, or personal opinions, but somehow quite of itself. Naturally only a numskull thinks of ghosts, but something like a primitive numskull thinks of ghosts but something like a primitive numskull seems to lurk beneath the surface of our reasonable daytime consciousness. (Jung, 1954, para. 512)

References

ABPS. (2015). What is black psychology? Retrieved from http://www.abpsi.org/pdf/ AfricanCenteredPsychologydefinition.Pdf

Abraham, N., & Torok, M. (1994). *The Shell and the Kernel.* Chicago, IL: University of Chicago Press.

Alexander, M. (2010). *The New Jim Crow: Mass incarceration in the area of color blindness.* New York, NY: The New Press.

Bollas, C. (1987). *The shadow of the object.* New York, NY: Columbia University Press.

Chomsky, N. (1968). *Language and mind.* New York, NY: Harcourt, Brace and World.

Coates, T.-N. (2015, October). The black family in the age of mass incarceration. *The Atlantic,* pp. 60–84.

Cox, R. (2015). *Where do we go from here? Mass Incarceration and the struggle for civil rights.* Executive Summary, Economic Policy Institute.

Freud, S. (1919). *The 'Uncanny'* (Collective Papers). New York, NY: Basic Books Inc., First American Edition, 1959.

Gordon, A. (1997). *Ghostly matters.* Minneapolis: University of Minnesota Press.

Grotstein, J. (2000). *Who is the dreamer who dreams the dream?* Hillsdale, NJ: Analytic Press.

Henderson, J. (1990). *Shadow and self.* Wilmette, IL: Chiron Press. 1990 p.103–113.

Jung, C. G. (1934/1954). *The development of personality.* New York, NY: Princeton University Press.

Jung, C. G. (1981) *The structure and dynamics of the psyche.* New York, NY: Princeton University Press.

Kimbles, S. (2000). The cultural complex and the myth of invisibility. In T. Singer (Ed.), *The vision thing: Myth, politics, and psyche in the world* (pp. 157–169). New York, NY: Routledge.

Kimbles, S. (2014). *Phantom narratives: The unseen contributions of culture to psyche.* Lanham, MD: Rowman & Littlefield.

Martinez, I. (2009). Toni Morrison's beloved: Slavery haunting America. *Journal of Jungian Scholarly Studies, 4*(3), 1–28.

Masschelein, A. (2011). *The unconcept.* Albany: State University of New York Press.

Morrison, T. (1987). *Beloved.* New York, NY: A Plume Book, Penguin Group.

Patterson, O. (1982). *Slavery and social death: A comparative study.* Cambridge: Harvard University Press.

Rahimi, S. (2013). The ego, the ocular, and the uncanny: Why are metaphors of vision central in accounts of the uncanny? *The International Journal of Psychoanalysis, 94,* 453–476.

Singer, T., & Kimbles, S. (Eds). (2004). *The cultural complexes. Contemporary perspectives on psyche and society.* New York, NY: Routledge.

Turner, V. (1966). *The ritual process: Structure and anti-structure.* New Brunswick, NJ: Aldine Transaction.

Engaging the anomalous: reflections from the anthropology of the paranormal

Jack Hunter

ABSTRACT

This review article looks at some of the parallels between the contents of this special issue on the paranormal and insights from the anthropology of religion, the anthropology of consciousness, transpersonal anthropology and the anthropology of the paranormal. The paper introduces the history of anthropology's engagement with the paranormal, from the early evolutionist perspectives of anthropology's pioneers to the most recent experiential approaches of the anthropology of consciousness. The paper concludes by highlighting the potential benefits of a cross-pollination of psychotherapeutic and anthropological research on the paranormal.

Das Anomale in Anspruch nehmen: Überlegungen aus Sicht der Anthropologie des Paranormalen

Dieser Übersichtsartikel nimmt einige inhaltliche Parallelen dieser Sonderausgabe zum Paranormalen und den Einsichten aus der Religions- und Bewusstseinsanthropologie sowie der transpersonalen als auch der paranormalen Anthropologie in den Blick. Der Artikel beginnt mit einem historischen Abriss zur Beschäftigung der Anthropologie mit dem Paranormalen, angefangen mit den Vorreitern der Anthropologie und deren evolutionstheoretischen Überlegungen, bis hin zu den neueren, empirischen Zugängen der Bewusstseinsanthropologie. Abschließend werden noch mögliche Vorteile aufgezeigt, die sich durch eine Verknüpfung von psychotherapeutischer und anthropologischer Forschungen zum Paranormalen erzielen ließe.

El compromiso con lo anómalo: Reflexiones de la antropología de lo paranormal

Este artículo crítico contempla algunos de los paralelos existentes entre los contenidos en este número especial acerca de lo paranormal y los diferentes puntos de vista de la antropología de la religión, la antropología de la conciencia, la antropología transpersonal y la antropología de lo paranormal. El artículo presenta la historia del compromiso de la antropología con lo paranormal, desde las perspectivas evolucionistas iniciales de sus fundadores hasta los métodos experienciales más recientes de la antropología de la conciencia. El artículo concluye destacando los beneficios potenciales de una polinización cruzada entre la antropología y la psicoterapia en la investigación de lo paranormal.

Ingaggiare l'anomalo: riflessioni relative all'antropologia del paranormale

Questa recensione esamina alcuni dei parallelismi tra i contenuti presenti in questo numero dedicato al paranormale e alcuni approfondimenti di antropologia della religione, antropologia della coscienza, antropologia transpersonale e antropologia del paranormale. Il contributo introduce alla storia del coinvolgimento dell'antropologia con il paranormale, dalle primi prospettive evoluzionistiche dei pionieri ddell'antropologia ai più recenti approcci esperienziali dell'antropologia della coscienza. L'articolo si conclude evidenziando i potenziali benefici di una "impollinazione incrociata" della ricerca psicoterapeutica e antropologica relativa al paranormale.

Solliciter l'anormalité: réflexions de l'anthropologie du paranormal

Cet article passe en revue certains des parallèles existant entre le contenu de ce numéro spécial sur le paranormal et une vision venant de l'anthropologie des religions, l'anthropologie de la conscience, l'anthropologie transpersonnelle et l'anthropologie du paranormal. L'article introduit l'histoire des relations entre anthropologie et paranormal, depuis les premières perspectives évolutionnistes des pionniers de l'anthropologie jusqu'aux approches anthropologiques de la conscience. L'article se termine par la mise en avant des bénéfices potentiels d'un enrichissement mutuel entre la recherche psychothérapeutique et la recherche anthropologique sur le paranormal.

Η ενασχόληση με το ανώμαλο: Σκέψεις από την Ανθρωπολογία του παραφυσικού

Αυτό το άρθρο ανασκόπησης εξετάζει μερικές από τις ομοιότητες μεταξύ του περιεχομένου αυτής της ειδικής έκδοσης για το παραφυσικό και των στοιχείων που προέκυψαν από την ανθρωπολογία της θρησκείας, την ανθρωπολογία της συνείδησης, τη διαπροσωπική ανθρωπολογία και την ανθρωπολογία του παραφυσικού. Το άρθρο παρουσιάζει την ιστορία της ενασχόλησης της ανθρωπολογίας με το παραφυσικό, από τις πρώτες εξελικτικές προοπτικές των πρωτοπόρων της ανθρωπολογίας μέχρι τις πιο πρόσφατες βιωματικές προσεγγίσεις της ανθρωπολογίας της συνείδησης. Καταλήγει τονίζοντας τα πιθανά οφέλη από μια διασταύρωση της ψυχοθεραπευτικής και ανθρωπολογικής έρευνας με το παραφυσικό.

I was very excited to hear that this special issue of the *European Journal of Psychotherapy and Counselling* was being put together, and was particularly honoured to have been invited to contribute a short reflection on its contents. Over the past several years, I have been actively involved in trying to initiate a similar dialogue in the context of my own discipline: anthropology. Indeed, there is a long and distinguished lineage to anthropology's engagement with the paranormal as a facet of human experience that goes right back to the discipline's nineteenth-century founders, though standard anthropology textbooks might not give any hint of this. Sir E.B. Tylor (1832–1917), for example, famous for his explanatory theory of 'animism' (the belief in spiritual beings as the most basic expression of religion), had investigated some of the leading Spiritualist mediums of his day. In spite of his clear interest in Spiritualism, however, Tylor never published accounts of his experiences, which included seances with the Reverend Stainton Moses (1839–1892), D.D. Home (1833–1896) and Kate Fox (1837–1892). Tylor's experiences only came to light following the researches of the historian of anthropology George W. Stocking Jr (1928–2013). In his private diaries, so Stocking discovered, Tylor admitted his bafflement at the strange things he had seen with these mediums, and came to the striking conclusion that there is a '*prima facie* case on evidence' for the abilities of certain mediums, and that 'there may be a psychic force causing raps, movements, levitations, etc.' (Stocking, 1971, pp. 92–100).

It is interesting to speculate on why Tylor decided against making his suspicions public, and a clue might be found in his own theory for the origin of animism. For Tylor, the belief in spirits arose out of misinterpretation, and in particular from mistaking dreams for reality. According to Tylor, who operated within a broadly evolutionist framework, so-called 'primitive' people developed the notion of spirits through failing to understand that the people they encountered in their dreams were not real, and from this misunderstanding went on to infer the existence of a non-physical part of the human that could leave the physical body under certain conditions, such as in trance, or in death (Tylor, 1930, p. 87). Belief in spirits, then, represented what Tylor called a 'survival,' something akin to a fossil of an outdated way of thinking, already superseded by rational and scientific modes of understanding the world. Tylor was a modern, rational, Victorian scholar, but he too had had unusual experiences in the presence of spirit mediums, experiences for which he could find no rational explanation. We might suggest, therefore, that Tylor's reluctance to publish his own paranormal experiences was, at least in part, due to the fact that to do so would be to admit that even the most distinguished, rational members of modern European societies can also have paranormal experiences. This would have been a direct challenge to the prevailing social-evolutionist paradigm of the time. It is also likely that Tylor was worried that an admission of even the possibility of a 'psychic force' could be detrimental to the emerging field of anthropology's status as a scientific discipline.

Tylor's example serves to illustrate two key points in discussions of the paranormal. Firstly, it highlights the fact that supernatural beliefs and paranormal experiences are *not* restricted to 'primitive' cultures, nor to non-Western societies. Indeed, they are surprisingly common within modern, post-industrial, Euro-American societies (Castro, Burrows, & Wooffitt, 2014). Secondly, it illustrates the problem that Euro-American academia (maybe even Euro-American culture as a whole) has with the so-called paranormal: it is taboo, not to be discussed or taken seriously. This is a problem that anthropology has long had to deal with, especially when anthropologists have been confronted with the belief systems and extraordinary claims of their fieldwork informants. The standard approach, following the lead of E.E. Evans-Pritchard (1902–1973), has since become a form of ontological bracketing. In his book *Theories of Primitive Religion* (1965), Evans-Pritchard writes:

> As I understand the matter, there is no possibility of knowing whether the spiritual beings of primitive religions or of any others have any existence or not, and since that is the case [the anthropologist] cannot take the question into consideration (Evans-Pritchard, 1965, p. 17)

This kind of approach has been immensely practical for anthropology, allowing it to document and describe a broad swathe of the world's cultures, and religious, magical and shamanistic belief systems, without the need to enter into debates about the reality status of the objects of such beliefs – this question is simply bracketed out. Things become a little less clear-cut, however, when anthropologists themselves begin to have experiences that seem to support the belief systems of their informants. How should such experiences be understood, and should they be included in ethnographic texts? Evans-Pritchard himself had such an experience while he conducted fieldwork amongst the Azande in Sudan. One night, while out for a walk, the anthropologist observed a mysterious light floating past his hut, seemingly on route to a nearby village. When he told his informants about the experience the next day, they immediately identified the light as 'witchcraft substance' on a murderous errand, and when a report arrived that an individual in the next village had died during the night, it further supported the Azande interpretation. In spite of this, however, Evans-Pritchard transforms the story into a joke in his monograph on Azande witchcraft beliefs, offering the suggestion that it was 'probably a handful of grass lit by someone on his way to defecate' (Evans-Pritchard, 1976, p. 11). Although clearly an advance of Tylor's approach to the paranormal, Evans-Pritchard still seems uncomfortable with admitting the possible reality of the paranormal.

A complete account of the development of transpersonal anthropology and the anthropology of consciousness exceeds the limitations of this short paper, but suffice to say at this juncture that it would be another forty or so years before anthropologists finally began to take heed of their own anomalous experiences in the field as potentially valuable research data, without attempting to reduce the complexity of the experience.[1] In the 1970s, two conferences specifically concerned with the implications of parapsychological research for anthropology were held in Mexico City and London, resulting in two ground-breaking publications (Angoff & Barth, 1974; Long, 1977). It was these conferences that ultimately paved the way for the emergence of the Society for the Anthropology of Consciousness, which is still very active today and has the stated aim of investigating 'psychic phenomena, reincarnation, near-near-death experiences, mediumistic communication, divination,' amongst other things (http://www.sacaaa.org/).

One of the leading lights in the anthropology of consciousness over the last 20 years has been Edith Turner, whose experience during the *Ihamba* healing ceremony of the Ndembu in Zambia was a major catalyst for her work on the experiential aspects of ritual healing (Turner, 1993). At the peak of the ritual, Turner witnessed the extraction of an amoprhic, plasma-like, grey blob from the back of an afflicted patient, she writes: 'a large gray blob about six inches across, a deep gray opaque thing emerging as a sphere. I was amazed – delighted. I still laugh with glee at the realisation of having seen it, the ihamba, and so big!' (Turner, 1998, p. 149). It was this sighting, amongst other experiences, that prompted Turner to conclude that anthropologists must learn to 'see as the Native sees' in order to understand ritual, and in doing so must:

> [...] endorse the experiences of spirits as veracious aspects of the life-world of the peoples with whom we work; that we faithfully attend to our own experiences in order to judge their veracity; that we are not reducing the phenomena of spirits or other extraordinary beings to something more abstract and distant in meaning; and that we accept the fact that spirits are ontologically real for those whom we study. (Turner, 2010, p. 224)

Turner's approach has been particularly influential in the anthropology of consciousness and the anthropology of religion in recent years, perhaps most notably in the work of Fiona Bowie, whose methodology of 'cognitive empathetic engagement' might be understood as a means of learning to 'see what the Native sees' in order to get at the underlying experiential core of religious, spiritual and paranormal belief and practice. Bowie explains how cognitive empathetic engagement requires the ethnographer to adopt 'the categories of his or her informants,' and to 'use this knowledge to interpret the world by means of those categories' as an 'effort of will and imagination.' Above all, the method requires 'an active engagement with another way of thinking, seeing and living' (Bowie, 2012, pp. 105–106).

Although much of this may seem tangential to the overall theme of this issue, in actuality, I think there are some rather striking correspondences. The case of E.B. Tylor, as well as the wider lineage of anthropology's involvement with the paranormal since its inception in the mid-nineteenth century, reveals a similar story to that outlined by Sommer in the paper 'Are You Afraid of the Dark?,' namely a contradictory fascination with the anomalous, paranormal and the occult in the development of modern science, coupled with an almost dogmatic desire to disenchant Euro-American academia, and to rid it of any hint of the magical. These same taboos are still in action today, ultimately resulting in a cultural fear of the anomalous, and an automatic association (and reduction) of anomalous experience to pathology. Examples from anthropology can show that this particular cultural framework is not the only one available for under-standing and working with anomalous experiences, and may prove useful for psychotherapists faced with clients reporting anomalous experiences.

E.B. Tylor's experience, and his unwillingness to talk about it in his published papers, also echoes Roxburgh and Evenden's article, 'They daren't tell people,' where we learn that those who have anomalous experiences often feel that they cannot talk about them for fear of 'being labelled with a mental disorder if they did' (Roxburgh and Evenden, this volume). Thankfully, things have changed since Tylor's day, and (some) anthropologists are now comfortable with owning up to their own anomalous experiences, encountered during their fieldwork, and are willing to explore their implications for ethnographic writing and theory formation. The same might also be said of psychotherapy and psychothera-pists. The wonderful book *Being Changed by Cross-Cultural Encounters* (1994) is a testament to this gradual shift in anthropology. It also hints at a breakdown of the usually assumed distinction between the observer and the observed. The anthropologist (perhaps also the psychotherapist) can no longer be thought of as somehow separate from the system they are investigating, they are also par-ticipants and their experiences matter too. Perhaps the anomalous experiences encountered by both anthropologists and psychotherapists can reveal insights into the life worlds of fieldwork informants and clients, respectively. See, as an example, Jokic's (2008) insights into Yanomamo cosmology revealed through his participation in shamanic ceremonies involving the psychoactive snuff *Yopo*.

Cameron's paper 'The Paranormal: An Unhelpful Concept in Psychotherapy and Counselling Research' also ties into all of this on two distinct fronts. Firstly, the author's conclusion that phenomenological bracketing represents the most fruitful means by which psychotherapists can accommodate the anomalous experiences of their clients seems to fall in line with Evans-Pritchard's approach of opting out of considering ontological questions, which is also the standard approach in disciplines such as anthropology and religious studies.[2] Secondly, the author's own anomalous experience of something resembling an 'elon-gated (and wriggly) jellybean: translucent, yet somehow also encased in with a slightly opaque shell' (Cameron, this volume), accords remarkably well with Edith Turner's experience during the *Ihamba* ceremony. This convergence poten-tially signals the centrality of anomalous experiences in the therapeutic setting (Turner's experience was, after all, also in the context of a healing ritual), and, as Cameron suggests, may indicate a need for psychotherapists to have an aware-ness of the research that has been conducted on anomalous experiences as part of their training (Cameron, this volume). This might also include an overview of the cross-cultural and ethnographic research on anomalous experiences and their role in traditional forms of shamanic healing (McClenon, 2001).

Kimbles argues that the concept of the 'Phantom Narrative,' as outlined in the paper 'Phantom Narratives and the Uncanny in Cultural Life,' 'operates in what Victor Turner ... has defined as a liminal space, which we might here speak of as a place between accepted cultural narrative' (Kimbles, this volume). Turner's notion of the liminal, derived from the earlier research of Arnold Van Gennep (1873–1957) on the structure of rituals, specifically in the context of rites of passage, has in recent years become a central focus in the anthropology of the paranormal. This emphasis has emerged largely from the work of the parapsychologist George Hansen, whose groundbreaking book *The Trickster and the Paranormal* (2001) suggests that paranormal manifestations are, by their very nature, liminal events. Hansen explains the central theme of his book:

> ... psi, the paranormal, and the supernatural are fundamentally linked to destructuring, change, transition, disorder, marginality, the ephemeral, fluidity, ambiguity, and the blurring of boundaries. (Hansen, 2001, 22)

From this perspective, then, the association between the paranormal and the psychotherapeutic process makes perfect sense. The psychotherapeutic process, like the shamanic healing ceremony, is a ritual, itself taking place within a liminal space separated from the outside world. It is also clear how, from this perspective, anomalous experiences might arise in individuals whose routine has been 'destructured,' who are in 'transition' or who feel 'marginalised.' The psychotherapeutic encounter, like the shamanic ritual, can help bring back order for the patient, help them make sense of their anomalous experiences, and eventually re-integrate themselves into society as part of the ritual structure.

To conclude, then, this special issue is a welcome contribution to the widening scholarly engagement with the anomalous, and I hope that some of the convergences I have highlighted, as preliminary as they are, might point to some interesting directions for future research. I am sure that anthropologists of the paranormal stand to learn a lot from the experiences of psychotherapists and their clients, and I am certain that the anthropological literature – particularly in the context of the anthropology of consciousness, transpersonal anthropology and paranthropology – contains valuable tools to help psychotherapists better make sense of anomalous experiences in their own practice.

Notes

1. For useful historical overviews of the development of transpersonal anthropology, the anthropology of consciousness and paranthropology, see: Schroll (2005), Luke (2010), Laughlin (2012), and Hunter (2012, 2015a).
2. I have argued elsewhere for an inversion of ontological bracketing, what I term 'ontological flooding' as a potential alternative approach to the paranormal. Instead of bracketing out ontological questions, we open the ontological floodgates and entertain a whole range of possibilities. In essence, this approach

destabilises ontological certainty, and opens up new avenues for research that the bracketed approach keeps shut (Hunter, 2015b). See also Northcote's (2004) paper on the limitations of bracketing in the investigation of supernormal claims.

References

Angoff, A., & Barth, D. (1974). *Parapsychology and anthropology: Proceedings of an international conference held in London, England, August 29–31, 1973.* New York, NY: Parapsychology Foundation.

Bowie, F. (2012). Devising methods for the ethnographic study of the afterlife: Cognition, empathy and engagement. In J. Hunter (Ed.), *Paranthropology: Anthropological approaches to the paranormal* (pp. 99–113). Bristol: Paranthropology.

Castro, M., Burrows, R., & Wooffitt, R. (2014). The paranormal is (still) normal: The sociological implications of a survey of paranormal experiences in great Britain. *Sociological Research Online, 18.*

Evans-Pritchard, E. E. (1965). *Theories of primitive religion.* Oxford: Clarendon Press.

Evans-Pritchard, E. E. (1976). *Witchcraft, oracles and magic among the azande.* Oxford: Clarendon Press.

Hansen, G. (2001). *The trickster and the paranormal.* Bloomington: X-Libris.

Hunter, J. (2012). *Paranthropology: Anthropological approaches to the paranormal.* Bristol: Paranthropology.

Hunter, J. (2015a). *Strange dimensions: A paranthropology anthology.* Llanrhaeadr-ym-Mochnant: Psychoid Books.

Hunter, J. (2015b). "Between Realness and Unrealness": Anthropology, parapsychology and the ontology of non-ordinary realities. *Diskus: Journal of the British Association for the Study of Religions, 17,* 4–20.

Jokic, Z. (2008). Yanomami shamanic initiation: The meaning of death and postmortem consciousness in transformation. *Anthropology of Consciousness, 19,* 33–59.

Laughlin, C. (2012). Transpersonal anthropology, then and now. In J. Hunter (Ed.), *Paranthropology: Anthropological approaches to the paranormal* (pp. 69–97). Bristol: Paranthropology.

Long, J. K. (1977). *Extrasensory ecology: Parapsychology and anthropology.* London: Scarecrow Press.

Luke, D. (2010). Anthropology and parapsychology: Still hostile sisters in science? *Time and Mind, 3,* 245–265.

McClenon, J. (2001). *Wondrous healing: Shamanism, human evolution and the origin of religion.* DeKalb: Northern Illinois University Press.

Northcote, J. (2004). Objectivity and the supernormal: The limitations of bracketing approaches in providing neutral accounts of supernormal claims. *Journal of Contemporary Religion, 19*, 85–98.

Schroll, M. A. (2005). Whither psi and anthropology? An incomplete history of SAC's origins, its relationship with transpersonal psychology and the untold stories of castaneda's controversy. *Anthropology of Consciousness, 16*, 6–24.

Stocking, G.W., Jr. (1971). Animism in theory and practice: E.B. Tylor's unpublished notes on "Spiritualism". *Man, 6*, 88–104.

Turner, E. (1993). The reality of spirits: A tabooed or permitted field of study?. *Anthropology of Consciousness, 4*, 9–12.

Turner, E. (1998). *Experiencing ritual: A new interpretation of African healing*. Philadelphia, PA: University of Pennsylvania Press.

Turner, E. (2010). Discussion: Ethnography as a transformative experience. *Anthropology and Humanism, 35*, 218–226.

Tylor, E. B. (1930). *Anthropology: An introduction to the study of man and civilization, II*. London: Watts & Co.

Young, D. E., & Goulet, J. G. (1994). *Being changed by cross-cultural encounters: The anthropology of extraordinary experience*. Ontario: Broadview Press.

The client, the therapist and the paranormal: a response

Tony R. Lawrence

ABSTRACT
In this paper, I provide a published paper response to the papers in this special edition on the paranormal and psychotherapy articulated largely from my career as a parapsychologist. In the introduction I note the definitional differences between advocates and counter-advocates in terms of what might be 'paranormal', although I argue ultimately that definitional differences aside, the therapist's relationship with the client's unusual experiences is critical, taking a phenomenological stance which is echoed by at least two of the papers in the special edition. In broad review, the papers make a variety of welcome contributions; historical individually and small sample phenomenological and also more metaphorically in terms of articulations of the haunting nature of collective and intergenerational trauma in the social and cultural sphere. I review the papers from a parapsychological perspective, considering the evidence drawn from parapsychological studies where it supports or adds to the topics of each paper. In concluding this response, it seems clear that therapists often work from first principles when relating to clients' anomalous experiences, and that the papers of the special edition each offer practising therapists some important evidential and practical insights into working with client presentations of ostensibly paranormal and anomalous experiences.

Der Klient, der Therapeut und das Paranormale: Eine Replik auf die Beiträge zur Sonderausgabe 'Psychotherapie und das Paranormale'

Mit diesem Artikel gebe ich eine Erwiderung auf die in dieser Sonderausgabe enthaltenen Beiträge zum Paranormalen innerhalb der Psychotherapie. Ich greife dabei weitestgehend auf meine Erfahrungen und Arbeiten als Parapsychologe zurück. Zu Beginn des Artikels gehe ich zunächst auf die definitorischen Unterschiede in Bezug auf das Paranormale von dessen Befürwortern aber auch Kritikern ein. Letzten Endes erachte ich diese unterschiedlichen Auffassungen abseits der Beziehung zwischen Therapeuten und Klienten, insbesondere auf Grundlage einer phänomenologischen Haltung, als problematisch – was meiner Meinung nach von mindestens zwei Beiträgen dieser Sonderausgabe transportiert wird. Im Großen und Ganzen jedoch liefern alle Artikel eine Reihe nützlicher Informationen; historisch betrachtet und anhand einiger phänomenologischer Beispiele, vor allem aber auf einer metaphorischen Ebene im Hinblick auf eine 'unheilvollen Natur' intergenerationaler und kollektiver Traumata in der gesellschaftlichen und kulturellen Sphäre. Ich nehme die Beiträge aus einer parapsychologischen Perspektive in den Blick und nehme gleichzeitig, soweit sinnvoll, für einige der Artikel Bezug auf aktuelle parapsychologische Studien. Zusammenfassend lässt sich feststellen, dass Therapeuten in Bezug auf anomale Erfahrungen von Klienten oftmals mit einigen Grundprinzipien reagieren. Hierzu liefern die Artikel dieser Sonderausgabe den Praktikern einige wichtige Informationen und Einblicke in die Arbeit mit Klienten und deren anscheinend anormalen bzw. paranormalen Erfahrungen.

El cliente, el terapeuta y lo paranormal: Una respuesta a la edición especial de psicoterapia y lo paranormal

En este artículo doy una respuesta a las diferentes ponencias en esta edición especial acerca de lo paranormal y la psicoterapia; mi respuesta corresponde a cómo he articulado el tema a través de mi carrera como parapsicólogo. En la introducción he notado diferencias en la definición entre los partidarios y los no partidarios en términos de lo que podría ser considerado como 'paranormal'. Se discute que las diferencias en definición, obviando la relación del terapeuta con las experiencias inusuales del cliente, es crítica al tomar una posición fenomenológica la encuentra eco en al menos dos de los artículos en esta edición especial. De una manera amplia los artículos presentan una variedad de contribuciones históricamente, individualmente, fenomenológicamente en menor grado y también metafóricamente, en términos de las relaciones de cómo se articula la inquietante naturaleza del trauma colectivo e intergeneracional en la esfera cultural y social. Se revisan los artículos desde la perspectiva parapsicológica, considerando la evidencia extraída de estudios parapsicológicos los cuales apoyan o agregan algo a los tópicos de cada artículo. Al concluir esta respuesta parece claro que los psicoterapeutas, frecuentemente trabajan apoyándose en ciertos principios en su relación con las experiencias anómalas de sus clientes y que cada artículo en esta edición especial ofrece a los terapeutas insights prácticos y evidentes para trabajar con clientes que presentan ostensiblemente experiencias paranormales y anómalas.

I cliente, il terapeuta e il Paranormale: una risposta alla Special Edition sulla psicoterapia e il paranormale

In questo lavoro cerco di fornire una risposta ai contributi proposti in questa special edition su paranormale e psicoterapia, risposta articolata in buona parte sulla mia esperienza come parapsicologo. Nell'introduzione rilevo le differenze nelle definizioni tra sostenitori ed oppositori rispetto a ciò che potrebbe essere 'paranormale' anche se io sostengo, in ultima analisi, che indipendentemente dalle differenze di definizione è fondamentale assumere una posizione fenomenologica, il che rimanda ad almeno un paio di contributi di questa edizione speciale. In senso ampio la lettura dei contributi presenta aspetti introduttivi, storie individualizzate e piccoli campioni fenomenologici, più metaforicamente una articolazione della natura del trauma collettivo e intergenerazionale in ambito sociale e culturale. Considero i contributi da una prospettiva parapsicologica, esaminando le evidenze tratte da studi parapsicologici che supportano o arricchiscono le argomentazioni di ogni contributo. Nel concludere, sembra chiaro che i terapeuti spesso lavorano a partire da principi fondamentali quando hanno a che fare con clienti che presentano esperienze anomale, inoltre ciascun contributi di questo numero offre importanti spunti pratici per il lavoro con clienti che presentano esperienze apparentemente paranormali e anomale.

Le client, le thérapeute et le paranormal: une réponse au numéro spécial sur la psychothérapie et le paranormal

Dans cet article je passe en revue les articles qui composent ce numéro spécial sur paranormal et psychothérapie et j'articule ma réponse aux articles à ma pratique de parapsychologue. Dans l'introduction je marque une différence définitionnelle entre les défenseurs et les pourfendeurs en termes ce qui pourrait être considéré comme 'paranormal' tout en argumentant qu'au final, différences définitionnelles mises à part, ce qui est essentiel c'est que la relation que le thérapeute a avec les expériences inhabituelles du client suive une attitude phénoménologique, ce qui est abordé dans au moins deux des articles de ce numéro spécial. De manière générale les articles fournissent une série d'heureuses contributions; historiquement, individuellement, à l'aide d'un petit échantillon quant à la recherche et phénoménologiquement mais également plus métaphoriquement en termes d'articulations entre la nature tourmentée du trauma collectif et intergénérationnel dans la sphère sociale et culturelle. Je passe en revue les articles avec une perspective parapsychologique, considérant les preuves apportées par les études parapsychologiques qui soutiennent ou ajoutent des éléments au propos de chaque article. Dans ma conclusion il apparaît clairement que les thérapeutes travaillent à partir de principes premiers lorsqu'ils sont en relation avec les expériences anomales des clients et que chacun des articles qui composent ce numéro spécial offre aux praticiens des preuves importantes et des perspectives pratiques pour le travail avec des clients présentant des expériences ostensiblement paranormales et anomales.

Ο Πελάτης, ο Θεραπευτής και το Παραφυσικό: Μια απάντηση στην Ειδική Έκδοση για την ψυχοθεραπεία και το παραφυσικό

Σε αυτό το άρθρο παρέχω μια δημοσιευμένη γραπτή απάντηση στα άρθρα της παρούσας ειδικής έκδοσης για το παραφυσικό και την ψυχοθεραπεία που βασίζεται σε μεγάλο βαθμό στην καριέρα μου ως παραψυχολόγου. Στην εισαγωγή σημειώνω τις διαφορές του ορισμού μεταξύ αυτών που τίθενται υπέρ και εναντίον του τι θα μπορούσε να είναι «παραφυσικό» παρόλο που υποστηρίζω τελικά ότι οι διαφορές στον ορισμό εκτός της σχέσης του θεραπευτή με την ασυνήθιστη εμπειρία του πελάτη αποτελούν περισσότερο μια φαινομενολογική στάση που αντανακλάται σε τουλάχιστον δύο από τα άρθρα στην ειδική έκδοση. Με μια γενική ματιά τα άρθρα προσφέρουν μια ποικιλία από συνεισφορές: ιστορικά διακεκριμένες, φαινομελογικές σε μικρό δείγμα και πιο μεταφορικά από την άποψη των διαρθρώσεων της στοιχειωμένης φύσης από συλλογικά και διαγενεακά τραύματα στον κοινωνικό και πολιτιστικό τομέα. Επανεξετάζω τα άρθρα από παραψυχολογική σκοπιά, λαμβάνοντας υπόψη τα στοιχεία που προέρχονται από παραψυχολογικές μελέτες όπου υποστηρίζεται ή προστίθεται στα θέματα του κάθε άρθρου. Συμπεραίνοντας, είναι σαφές ότι οι θεραπευτές συχνά δουλεύουν με τα στοιχειώδη, όταν συνδέονται με πελάτες με ανώμαλες εμπειρίες, και ότι τα άρθρα της ειδικής έκδοσης προσφέρουν στους ασκούμενους θεραπευτές κάποιες σημαντικές εμπειρικές και πρακτικές γνώσεις για να εργάζονται με πελάτες που παρουσιάζουν φαινομενικά παραφυσικές και ανώμαλες εμπειρίες.

While Freud was going on this way, I had a curious sensation. It was as if my diaphragm were made of iron and were becoming red-hot – a glowing vault. And at that moment there was such a loud report in the bookcase, which stood right next to us, that we both started up in alarm, fearing the thing was going to topple over on us. I said to Freud: 'There, that is an example of a so-called catalytic exteriorisation phenomenon'.

'Oh come', he exclaimed. 'That is sheer bosh'.

'It is not', I replied. 'You are mistaken, Herr Professor. And to prove my point I now predict that in a moment there will be another loud report!'

Sure enough, no sooner had I said the words than the same detonation went off in the bookcase … Freud stared aghast at me. (Jung, 1983, pp. 178, 179)

Introduction

For someone who has a PhD in Parapsychology (Lawrence, 1998), and who is presently training to become a psychotherapist, the invitation to provide a published response to this special edition of the EJCP on psychotherapy and the paranormal felt both welcome and almost synchronistic. Having spent much of my late teens moving from a position of naive wonder about the paranormal to eventually completing my PhD in parapsychology at the Koestler Parapsychology Research Unit under the supervision of Professor Robert Morris, to finding myself now engaged in the end-stage business of training for a second career in the world of psychotherapy, I found myself wondering which of two hats I should wear in writing my response to the papers of this special edition. I decided, ultimately, to wear both hats when reading the papers that comprise this special edition, with some personal acknowledgement that I have worn the parapsychological hat for longer!

The quote with which I start this response to the papers in the special edition cuts straight to so many of the themes which the authors of the various papers presented; that the early psychotherapists were interested in that class of human experiences we commonly term 'paranormal', that opinions could be strongly divided between the sceptic and the believer, and that whatever position one did take on such phenomena, their intrusion into the normative course of mundane existence demands some kind of inquiry. Whether or not one believes that paranormal phenomena are 'real' (whatever that might mean), they are indefatigable experiences which seem to have a perennial presence within human experience. As such, it is inevitable that psychotherapists might come across client accounts of such experiences in their career.

One of the sometimes implicit and sometimes explicit issues represented in the papers presented in the special edition is what the term paranormal denotes. As someone who has worked actively as an academic parapsychologist, I have elsewhere argued (Lawrence, 2001) that the term paranormal most clearly denotes '... hypothesized processes that in principle are physically impossible or outside the realm of human capabilities as presently conceived by conventional scientists ...'[1] Thus for the parapsychologist, the common realm of experiences which are the focus of investigation are, broadly but not exhaustively, as follows; telepathy (seemingly direct apprehension of the mental experiences of another human being), clairvoyance (seemingly direct apprehension of objective events in the world without apparent mediation and communication from the mind of another person), precognition (seemingly direct apprehension of the future),[2] psychokinesis (the seeming ability of the mind to influence the physical world – or as Jung in the quote starting this published response would have called it the 'catalytic exteriorisation phenomenon'), out-of-body experiences (e.g. Alvarado, 2000), near-death experiences, cases suggestive of reincarnation, mediumistic phenomena (Braude, 2003; Gauld, 1982), and apparitions and poltergeist phenomena (e.g. Gauld & Cornell, 1979; Houran & Lange, 2001).

The clear thread running through all of these phenomena is that (a) they happen to human beings and (b) if convincingly demonstrated to be 'real' they would significantly extend our understanding of human capability (as the subtitle of one of the main 'textbooks' of parapsychology clearly indicated; Edge, Morris, Palmer, & Rush, 1986). However, it is worth noting that outside of parapsychology, the term paranormal may be used more loosely; for example, sceptics (e.g. Tobacyk & Milford, 1983) tend towards a view of the paranormal which also includes such things as bigfoot, aliens and UFOs, and common or garden superstitious beliefs. I myself regard the distinction between the terms 'anomalous' and 'paranormal' as helpful in demarcating what it is that parapsy-chologists are interested in; all so-called 'paranormal' phenomena are indeed examples of 'anomalous' phenomena, but not all 'anomalous' phenomena are paranormal (at least as I or most parapsychologists would define that term). Anomalous phenomena are for me, reasonably defined as phenomena of any kind which fail to sit within some conventional or scientifically given lawful understanding of nature. Anomalous phenomena may therefore be well within, as well as outwith, ordinary or conventional science.

Regardless, as I read through the papers in the special edition, I found that I was not concerned so much with strict definitions of the paranormal, the anom-alous, or indeed (with a nod to my psychodynamic colleagues the 'uncanny'), but felt that ultimately there is merit in simply considering what therapeutically might be the stance to take with respect to this class of client experiences what-ever the precise terminology we choose. In responding to the special edition papers, I shall in what follows consider each paper in turn, and it seems appro-priate to begin my response with the paper dealing with matters of historical concern.

Are you afraid of the dark?

Whether I read this paper by Sommer with my parapsychologist's hat on or my trainee psychotherapist's hat on, I found this essentially historical evaluation of the relationship between belief and disbelief in the paranormal engaging and stimulating. As Sommer is at pains to point out, a historical examination of the early days of psychology clearly demonstrates a more diverse position amongst early psychologists with respect to the issue of the paranormal. From my own experience of teaching the early history of academic psychology, it was already apparent to me that the triple influences of mesmerism (now hypnotism), spirit-ualism and phrenology provided a fertile social and popular cultural milieu for raising awareness of evidential issues relating to the human mind/spirit (see e.g. Benjamin, 2006).

Sommer presents the view that historical examination of interest and attitudes towards the paranormal amongst the early founders of psychology reveals many complexities in those attitudes, and that any modern-day attempt to polarize such issues as being solely about replacing the pre-enlightenment values of religious and superstitious thinking with those of enlightenment rationality and empiricism is a myth. Moreover, in the section of the paper on the 'Will to believe', Sommer gives well overdue attention to the possibility that a more intimate acquaintance with the history of psychology might establish an equally strong case for a 'will to disbelieve'. Here I might merely note that in my own PhD research which related to the literature on the psychology of paranormal belief, I could find a great many empirical studies which explicitly focused on the factors which predispose people to believe in the paranormal but almost nothing where the focus was on factors which predispose people to disbelieve. To the extent therefore that one wanted to build an understanding of the psychology of *scepticism,* it must largely be done by implicit inference rather than direct explicit results of studies focused on the basis for scepticism. Thus, Sommer's suggestion that the grounds for sceptical disbelief might not always have resided in the enlightenment values of rationalism and hard-nosed empiricism, but themselves often contain pointers towards irrationality, emotionality and rhetorically driven polemicism in making way for a 'proper' science of psychology are well made, and for readers who are interested in examining the early history of psychical research to capture the same sense of the value of detailed and nuanced historical account of the formation of that field, I would strongly recommend Gauld's (1968) book, 'The Founders of Psychical Research'.

In parallel, the transition from psychical research to the modern field of parapsychology, carried *within* the field a turn towards a more scientifically positioned, lab-based, experimental approach to investigation of the paranormal, where the establishment of scientifically acceptable proof of paranormal phenomena through laboratory experiments capable of being statistically demonstrated became the abiding legacy of the principle founder of the modern field of parapsychology, Joseph Banks Rhine. However, as Cameron argues, the terms of evidence and debate that Rhine set up for the modern field of parapsychological investigation of the paranormal, which still exert a strong influence upon parapsychology to this day, might not be ones which therapists need to articulate with in the therapy room.

The paranormal: an unhelpful concept in psychotherapy and counselling

The presentation in this paper of a real exchange between the author (as therapist) and the client, and the subsequent essentially phenomenological rather than metaphysical orientation towards the felt and practical relational meaning of the experience, offers a concrete orientation to the presence of one experiential encounter that might be termed uncanny, deeply intuitive or indeed paranormal. However, as Cameron makes strongly and emphatically clear, in the therapeutic relationship, the question of the intrinsic reality of the paranormal is not helpful and I felt strongly inclined to agree.

For Cameron, the 'bizarre' perceptual occurrence of the jelly-bean, and the attendant intuitive feelings of disappointment, offer the opportunity to consider the split between essentially metaphysical considerations that are likely to lead nowhere with the client – questions about how the jelly-bean articulates with the therapist's or client's conventional sense of reality – or the much more productive turn towards the lived experience in its whole cloth phenomenological character. In being with the whole experience in that moment of relating with the client, the author reports merely noting the passing oddity and unusualness of the jelly-been 'image' itself though not getting caught up with it, but also is able to experience the sense of heartfelt disappointment somehow connected to the quasi-visual jelly-bean hovering over her client's chest. After a period of intuitive consideration of the sense of disappointment, the therapist feels moved to share, not so much the originating perception of the wriggly bean, but the felt sense of disappointment so closely connected with it. As it happens what is shared proves to be highly appropriate for the client, and moves the client forward in their experiencing of their problem with their manager and indeed opens up new territory on the broader topic of feeling let down in life for the client to share with the therapist.

In the remainder of the paper, the author offers a consideration of parapsychology partly in terms of useful historical content drawing largely upon Beloff (1993), but in particular focusing on Collins and Pinch's (1979) insightful sociological examination of the marginalization of the science of parapsychology by mainstream science. Certainly in my career as a parapsychologist, I found that there was an almost uniform assumption of the pseudo-scientific nature of parapsychology amongst 'armchair' sceptics and many (though not all) mainstream psychological colleagues, but at the Koestler Parapsychology Research Unit where I completed my PhD, Professor Morris tended towards an open and dialogical stance towards both issues of advocacy and counter-advocacy of the study of the paranormal, and to the extent that certain prominent sceptical commentators visited the Koestler Parapsychology Unit, my sense during my time there (1992–1996) was that they realized that parapsychologists were open-minded folks pursuing their interests as scientifically and rationally as our mainstream psychological colleagues.

The ending section of this paper presented a sound phenomenological underpinning for the experience recounted and overall, whether I read the paper as a parapsychologist or a psychotherapist, I was in complete agreement with the conclusion that therapists need to relate to what is experienced in the therapeutic encounter with the client, rather than in terms of what might happen in parapsychological experiments. Interestingly, this same practical sense of staying with the client's experiences and meanings in an exploratory and phenomenologically inclined manner proved to be an important finding of the next paper by Roxburgh and Evenden.

They daren't tell the people

I found the paper by Roxburgh and Evenden to be very informative indeed. Whereas the previous paper by Cameron focuses on a single encounter between therapist and client, in which the therapist experiences something unusual, the authors of this paper conducted a strong qualitatively oriented thematic analysis of a sample of therapists' encounters with 'anomalous experiences'. In their introduction to their research, Roxburgh and Evenden quite comprehensively outline the growth of interest in anomalous experiences amongst mental health clinicians generally, and from this review it does indeed seem appropriate to refer to the development of a fledgling field of clinical parapsychology. One of the things that stood out for me in the introduction was the tension between those such as Hastings (1983), who advocates developing reality tests for the genuineness of client anomalous experiences, versus those such as Parra (2012), who argue resonantly with Cameron that it is not the role of therapists to authenticate the client's experience – once again touching upon the deeper tension between metaphysical and phenomenological 'authenticity' of client experience.

In terms of the sample of therapist participants for this thematic analysis, it was good to see a reasonable range of modalities presented, and especially good to see that a CBT therapist was amongst the participants (a notable omission amongst the submitted papers in this special edition I feel). I found myself wondering whether the relatively large subsample of transpersonally oriented therapists might influence the study outcomes – transpersonal psychology (which I have myself taught) very naturally embraces a wide range of spiritual or spiritual-type experiences, but it remains for future research of this kind to establish whether the thematic findings of this particular study are reliably indicated amongst a broader, possibly more demographically representative range of therapists. This gentle caution (shared to be fair by the authors) aside, the themes found are of considerable interest, and go a long way I feel to meeting the authors' desire to 'redress the gap' in the UK-based research on therapists' work with clients who report anomalous experiences.

The theme of 'testing the waters' points to the clearly demonstrated experience of stigma that clients might attach to self-disclosing their anomalous experiences. Even in my purely parapsychological career, if I was contacted by members of the public I often found that it took a little time reassuring them that I didn't think they were 'mad' before the individual would more fully disclose the richness of their anomalous experiences. Given that clients who see therapists are individuals who experience mental vulnerability of some kind, there is clearly potential for a double stigma amongst those clients whose experiences also include encounters with the anomalous or ostensibly paranormal. Indeed, the presence of this theme very strongly underlined for me the importance of therapists taking an intrinsically phenomenological and non-judgemental stance towards the client's experience of the anomalous – I certainly feel it is unlikely that clients would disclose such experiences if they felt that such experiences would be subjected to a 'reality test' (however well intentioned), and indeed the second theme only bolsters this conclusion.

The second theme of 'exploration not explanation' revealed that for this group of therapists, any tendency to relate to the client's anomalous experience from the therapist's own frame of reference was to be avoided. Once again, staying with the exploration of the client's experience, however odd it may appear to the therapist was the preferred option indicated in the excerpts quoted by four of the therapists. This theme gave me pause for thought in terms of something the authors raised in both the introduction and the discussion, and again in the third theme of 'special but not unique' – the issue of 'normalizing' the client's experience of the anomalous. On the one hand, normalization has the beneficial task of (potentially) letting clients know that their experience is shared with others and is not so 'strange'. But I could imagine quite easily that for some clients with anomalous experiences, any knee-jerk or unsolicited attempt by the therapist at 'normalizing' might be contra-indicated; for example, in the case of the client for whom the experiencing of anomalous events strongly represents a specialness or uniqueness of self, or for whom the experience is deeply connected in some network of meanings that ultimately are inseparable from the client's more mundane experiences. It seemed to me that if the therapist stays closely and empathically within the clients' core anomalous experience(s) and their associated network of attendant meanings and values in a tentative and exploratory way, then this exploratory sensitivity to the place of the anomalous experience within the whole person of the client is more likely to lead to nuances in the therapist's working with normalization of client anomalous experience (or not as the case may be).

The fourth and final theme of 'forewarned and forearmed' spoke expressly to the therapists sense of how UK therapists presently seemed left to their own devices in articulating the relationship with clients' experience of the anomalous. In addition, given this is clearly the case, it is suggested that psychotherapy training programmes might benefit from some orientation to anomalous experiences in client work. Whether this occurs in the context of initial training or in terms of post-training continuing professional development workshops, it struck me that, in many respects, the therapists in this study raise a very valid prospect. To this end, I would recommend the excellent book edited by Cardeňa, Lynn, and Krippner (2000) as a well-edited source of highly readable chapters covering a good range of anomalous experiences, written by leading experts in the field. It is the kind of book that would certainly meet the study authors' suggestion in the discussion that therapists, services and training organizations have'… adequate and reliable information about AEs …'. Quite generally, I found that the authors' discussion articulated very well with the issues raised in the study, and contained many important suggestions for directions future research might take.

Phantom narratives

A very interesting, but perhaps for me somewhat problematic, paper in this special issue on the paranormal and psychotherapy, was the paper on 'Phantom Narratives'. I found the paper interesting because it proposes that phantom narratives are psychic[3] presences that exist at the interface of personal affect and experience, on the one hand, and the traumas of social, historical and cultural marginalization and disempowerment, on the other. However, I found myself entirely split in my responses to the paper between my older identity as a parapsychologist, and my greener one as a trainee psychotherapist. I shall explain.

With my parapsychologist's hat on I, through successive readings, found that I could not quite shake off the sense that the terms 'phantom', 'phantomatic', 'psychic', 'presences', 'uncanny', 'haunting' were being used as artful metaphors for essentially worldly individual and group dynamics of marginalization, social and political repression, and the traumas of cultural invisibility that result, and in this regard I found the paper of perhaps at best tangential relevance to the context of usage of the term paranormal with which this special edition is more directly focused. However, this being said, in dealing with themes of marginalization and intergenerational trauma, I could at least see that the paper touches, unwittingly but relevantly, on issues which have exercised the theoretical imaginations of some psychologists who have investigated the possible causes of paranormal belief. For example, one of three major theories of the origination of paranormal belief has been what might be termed the 'Social Marginality' Theory (see e.g. Bainbridge, 1978; Wuthnow, 1976). Those who propose this view argue that paranormal beliefs are indeed taken on precisely because those adopting them have a marginal social status. I have elsewhere offered a concise review of the evidence for and against this view in Lawrence (2001), but as I concluded at the time there is, once the evidence is reviewed, little clear-cut direct evidence for the view that social marginalization leads *directly* to paranormal belief.

However, in my own PhD thesis (Lawrence, 1998; but see also Lawrence, Edwards, Barraclough, Church, & Hetherington, 1995), I investigated the childhood causes and consequences of paranormal belief and experience, and in that more psychologically and individually oriented set of studies, I did find much support for the notion that traumatic events in childhood are significantly related to subsequent adult self-report levels of both paranormal experience and paranormal belief. In particular, I found that there were two likely causal routes for the influence of childhood trauma on adult paranormal experience and belief; one was a direct influence of loss-related trauma upon paranormal experience (e.g. the death of a parent in childhood might be directly associated with a paranormal experience), whilst the second route was that of control-related trauma which was indirectly related to paranormal experience and belief via the mediating influence of childhood fantasy (e.g. sexual, physical and emotional abuse in childhood tended to relate directly to the early childhood development of imaginative fantasy as a means of coping with such trauma, and the heightened imaginative/fantasy-prone orientation fostered by chronic coping through fantasy in childhood was itself then directly related to paranormal experience, though interestingly *not* to paranormal belief). Thus, there is a role for childhood trauma in understanding the formation of paranormal belief and experience, and obviously trauma rarely springs *de novo* into the life of families – traumatizing parents and caregivers are themselves often victims of trauma in their own earlier lives. I do not doubt then that at some level intergenerational trauma does have an impact upon the likelihood of experiencing and believing in the paranormal (especially experiencing).

Parapsychological considerations aside, when I read the paper on phantom narratives with a purely psychotherapist's hat on, I found it offered a stimulating psychodynamic account of the interface between consciousness and unconsciousness in respect of concepts drawn and inspired by the author's Jungian psychotherapeutic orientation, and its metaphors of phantomatic presence resonated with my sense of the author's passion for the collective unfinished business that results from social, cultural, economic and political marginalization.

Conclusion

As Roxburgh and Evenden discovered in this special edition, therapists working with clients' anomalous experiences in the therapy room (at least in the UK but I largely suspect worldwide) often end up having to work from therapeutic first principles, without recourse to the full range of evidence relating to sober, open-minded and seriously intentioned investigation (whether quantitative or qualitative, or by advocate or counter-advocate) of the nature of such experiences. My strong sense in concluding this response to the papers of the special edition on the paranormal and psychotherapy is that papers of this kind are of the utmost importance in stimulating and facilitating the therapist's capacity to relate with client expressions of the anomalous.

Notable by its absence (for the greatest part) was any paper submission on the relationship between cognitive-behavioural therapy and clients' anomalous experiences. It seems to me that of all the mainline therapeutic modalities, the cognitive-behavioural therapists' response to anomalous client experiences would be most intriguing, though also most welcome. Perhaps the papers of the special edition will stimulate contributions from the CBT community of therapists at some later stage.

But in closing, I very much hope that readers of the special edition share with me and the fellow authors of the papers presented, an enhanced sense that a greater engagement with the wider historical, sociocultural, psychological and indeed parapsychological evidence base of anomalous experiences can enable (most importantly for therapists) a more informed and active phenomenological exploration of anomalous experiences in the relational space between the client and therapist. Whatever hat I wore when reading the presented papers, I personally and professionally have no doubt that this is of great value in enabling the therapist to further the client's own engagement therapeutically with the boundaries of self, world and other, however blurred, anomalous, uncanny or indeed paranormal those boundaries may sometimes seem.

Notes

1. This definition is not originally mine, but is used also by Irwin (1993), who bases it on Thalbourne (1982).
2. These three, plus psychokinesis, are often termed more generally 'Psi' by parapsychologists. The trio of telepathy clairvoyance and precognition are often generally labelled 'Extra Sensory Perception' (ESP).
3. Of course, the term 'psychic' means largely different things to the parapsychologist, on the one hand, and the psychodynamic therapist, on the other, although I felt implicitly that the sense intended by Kimbles was more nearly the latter one. Indeed, precisely, this conflation of psychic-paranormal and psychic-of-the-psyche, hampered my efforts to integrate the split I felt in considering the relevance of the paper to the direct issue of the psychic *qua* paranormal.

References

Alvarado, C. (2000). Out-of-body experiences. In E. Cardeña, S. J. Lynn, & S. Krippner (Eds.), *Varieties of anomalous experience: Examining the scientific evidence* (pp. 183–218). Washington, DC: American Psychological Association.

Bainbridge, W. S. (1978). Chariots of the gullible. *Skeptical Inquirer, 3*, 33–48.

Beloff, J. (1993). *Parapsychology: A concise history*. London: Athlone Press.

Benjamin, L. T. (2006). *A brief history of modern psychology*. Oxford: Blackwell.

Braude, S. E. (2003). *Immortal remains*. Oxford: Rowman and Littlefield.

Cardeña, E., Lynn, S. J., & Krippner, S. (2000). *Varieties of anomalous experience: Examining the scientific evidence*. Washington, DC: American Psychological Association.

Collins, H. M., & Pinch, T. J. (1979). The construction of the paranormal: Nothing unscientific is happening. In R. Wallis (Ed.), *On the margins of science: The social construction of rejected knowledge* (pp. 237–270). Keele: Sociological Review Monograph 27.

Edge, H. L., Morris, R. L., Palmer, J., & Rush, J. H. (1986). *Foundations of parapsychology: Exploring the boundaries of human capability*. London: Routledge and Kegan Paul.

Gauld, A. (1968). *The founders of psychical research*. London: Routledge and Kegan Paul.

Gauld, A. (1982). *Mediumship and survival: A century of investigation*. London: Heinemann.

Gauld, A., & Cornell, A. (1979). *Poltergeists*. London: Routledge and Kegan Paul.

Hastings, A. (1983). A counseling approach to parapsychological experience. *Journal of Transpersonal Psychology, 15*, 143–167.

Houran, J., & Lange, R. (2001). *Hauntings and apparitions: Multi-disciplinary perspectives*. Jefferson, NC: McFarland.

Irwin, H. J. (1993). Belief in the paranormal: A review of the empirical literature. *Journal of the American Society for Psychical Research, 87*, 1–39.

Jung, C. G. (1983). *Memories, dreams, reflections*. London: Fontana.

Lawrence, T. R. (1998). *The childhood causes and consequences of paranormal belief and experience* (Unpublished PhD thesis). Edinburgh: University of Edinburgh.

Lawrence, T. R. (2001). Apparitions and kindred phenomena: Their relevance to the psychology of paranormal belief and experience. In J. Houran & R. Lange (Eds.), *Hauntings and apparitions: Multi-disciplinary perspectives* (pp. 248–259). Jefferson, NC: McFarland.

Lawrence, T. R., Edwards, C., Barraclough, N., Church, S., & Hetherington, F. (1995). Modelling childhood causes of paranormal belief and experience: Childhood trauma and childhood fantasy. *Personality and Individual Differences, 19*, 209–215.

Parra, A. (2012). Group therapy approach to exceptional human experiences: An Argentinean experience. In W. H. Kramer, E. Bauer, & G. H. Hövelmann (Eds.), *Perspectives of clinical parapsychology: An introductory reader* (pp. 88–102). Bunnik: Stichting Het Johan Borgman Fonds.

Thalbourne, M. A. (1982). *A glossary of terms used in parapsychology*. London: Heinemann.

Tobacyk, J. J., & Milford, G. (1983). Belief in paranormal phenomena: Assessment instrument development and implications for personality functioning. *Journal of Personality and Social Psychology, 44*, 1029–1037.

Wuthnow, R. (1976). Astrology and marginality. *Journal for the Scientific Study of Religion, 15*, 157–168.

The magic of the relational

Del Loewenthal

There is a growing interest in relational therapy (Greenberg & Mitchell, 1983; Mitchell & Aron, 1999; Safran & Muran, 2000) as well as research on relating in psychotherapy (Birtchnell, 1999) and relational research (Loewenthal, 2007). For some, the relational is most apparent in the psychoanalytic traditions of Freud, Klein and object relations theories as well as Jung; however, the increased interest in relational psychotherapy also includes a whole range of humanistic, existential, integrative and other approaches (see for example Loewenthal & Samuels, 2014).

Importantly there is growing international recognition, of what is taken as research evidence (Beutler & Harwood, 2002; Luborsky & Auerbach, 1985), which suggests it is the relationship that is the most important factor in facilitating a successful outcome in psychological therapy. Furthermore, following the pioneering work of those such as Stephen Mitchell (1988), there is the emergence of organisations such as The International Association for Relational Psychoanalysis and Psychotherapy.

But what then, of the different theories in psychological therapies, regarding questions of 'the relational'? Do they make any difference, for example, do notions of object relations help or hinder? Is relational psychoanalysis really any different? Does the notion of learning relational skills just lead to further alienated inauthenticity in the name of authenticity? How can it be that, for some, interpreting the transference is a form of persecutory violence, whereas, for others, it's an ethical responsibility? Does naming a therapeutic modality as relational increase the possibility of a more human and fruitful approach or is it really an inappropriate, unhelpful demand from the therapist, brought about from what is lacking in the therapist's own life? So, is it helpful to link psychotherapy with the name 'relationa'? In particular, isn't there a danger of putting characteristics to the word 'relationship' and making it a technology where we talk about the 'relational', 'relationality', and so forth? Perhaps Heidegger's (1962) 'being with' is one alternative, if one could then stop it becoming a technology.

Yet, what I hesitantly term 'relational learning' does seem to have vital intrinsic qualities. How many readers' favourite and their children's favourite school subjects have consistently changed as their teachers have changed?

What is it then about the relationship that makes the difference? Perhaps it's magic! Whatever it is, perhaps it needs to remain mysterious – for as Merleau-Ponty (1956) wrote, once you take away the mystery, you can take away the thing itself.

Does potentially Polanyi's (2009) 'Tacit knowledge' come closest to describing what happens through the relational in therapy? If so, it is not something that can be taught and learned by either trainee psychological therapists or patients/clients. But might it be imparted and acquired? So, should we attempt a definition of the relational (with reification apologies), or does its tacit, perhaps magical qualities make this too problematic? Hargaden and Schwartz (2007), who edited one of the two special issues of the *European Journal of Psychotherapy and Counselling* from which this chapter has evolved, identify what they consider to be key elements of relational psychotherapy:

- The centrality of the relationship
- Therapy as a two-way street involving a bidirectional process
- Both the vulnerability of therapist and client are involved
- Countertransference is used, not merely as information but in thoughtful disclosure and collaborative dialogue
- The co-construction and multiplicity of meaning

Hargaden and Schwartz (2007) suggest that relational psychoanalysis usually tends to be regarded as a distinctive contemporary American contribution to psychoanalysis, emanating from the interpersonal (Washington) school of psychoanalysis associated with the psychiatrists Harry Stack Sullivan and William Alanson White. White in particular was instrumental, in the 1920s, in questioning the classical Freudian perspective, insisting that psychosis was capable of being treated psychodynamically with Freud's techniques. In the 1970s, a group of analysts (including Stephen Mitchell and Jay Greenberg at the William Alanson White Institute in New York) began to explore extensions of Sullivan's interpersonal psychoanalysis and what has become known as relational psychoanalysis emerged from this grouping.

Hargaden and Schwartz (2007) contend, however, that the relational perspective has in fact deep European roots that began with Eugen Bleuler, at the Rheinau Hospital for the Insane just outside Strasbourg. Bleuler maintained the possibility of relating to and understanding the utterances of the deeply disturbed people that he was to call schizophrenic. Hargaden and Schwartz (2007) see the tension between instinctual and relational approaches to mental distress as inherent in Freud's writings and additionally, the work of Donald Winnicott, Ronald Fairbairn and John Bowlby are viewed as central to object relations and attachment theory – a development in Europe closely intertwining with the developing relational approaches in the US.

There is the belief that there are significant humanistic routes to relational psychoanalysis (Hargaden & Schwartz, 2007) including the work of Carl
Rogers. Two films entitled *The Right to Be Desperate* and *Anger and Hurt* show
Rogers working with a man who was very ill and a victim of racism. In these
films, Rogers works with a deep concentrated listening that is described as
benign, yet intense and with a great warmth and depth of intellect. Hargaden
and Schwartz (2007) regard this type of listening as very skilled and deeply
empathic, whilst also retaining the therapist's subjective sense of self. This is
viewed as the essence of a relational approach to working with clients.

If we then think that as psychological therapists we can actually be helpful,
focusing on relationships, what are we actually looking at relationships
between? Following Malan (1999), we might think it is the relationship
between the patient/client and the psychological therapist; and/or the relationship between the patient/client and those around the client; and/or relationship between the patient/client and significant others in their past.

However, if we were to return to William James (1890), a founding father of
psychology, (which psychologists, never mind psychotherapists, might benefit
in reading), one would find he speaks about relationships in three different
ways: first, between things, which would include the relationships between
person and persons – this is 'intersubjectivity'. Yet, what is intersubjectivity? Is
it not magic? But isn't it a kind of magic which objective thinking cannot reach,
for to quote Kierkegaard:

> While objective thought is indifferent to the thinking subject and his existence,
> the subjective thinker is an existing individual interested in his own thinking,
> existing as he does in his thought. His thinking has therefore a different type of
> reflection, namely the reflection of inwardness, of possession, by virtue of which
> it belongs to the thinking subject and to no one else. While objective thought
> translates everything into results, and helps all mankind to cheat, by copying
> these off and reciting them by rote, subjective thought puts everything in pro-
> cess and omits the result: partly because this belongs to him who has the way,
> and partly because as an existing individual he is constantly in process of coming
> to be, which holds true of any human being who has not permitted himself to be
> deceived into becoming objective. (Kierkegaard, 1941: 67)

Thus, as argued in Loewenthal (2017), psychotherapy here could be seen
to be not about goals or notions of objective reality but more about how
patients/clients view their world in their striving for existence.

But to return to James (1890) his other two relationships are: the relations
between persons and their materiality and environment (termed 'inter-
materiality') and third, what I would like also to briefly explore here: the relationship between person and method (called 'intermethodology').

So, what may be particularly important is the relationship between the psychological therapist and their particular mode of working. For different modes
of working probably (seemingly magically) evoke thoughts, feelings and

behaviours of different orders. What James (1912) attempted to knock on the head was the traditional belief that methods usage only implicates the intellect by stating that passion, taste, emotion and practice cooperate in science as much as in any other practical affair. This radical empiricism is in contrast to the traditional belief that method functions independently of the total personalities who use them. This raises such questions as the potential suitability of the individual psychological therapist to carry out a particular therapeutic approach, as well as the effect of the professional training on the person.

With ideas of radical empiricism, developed from James, what is being suggested here is, first an interest in the relationship of the person who is the psychological therapist with the particular method/school of psychotherapy they have chosen and what qualities it brings out in the therapist that are helpful and unhelpful for the therapeutic endeavour. Second, there is the question as to what else the particular modality method allows, perhaps despite itself, to percolate through beyond its self-contained, detached, professional posturing. Here, we might see what the spaces between our method give rise to. In the case of psychological therapies, we attempt to give names to what happens in such spaces such as 'transference' and 'countertransference', 'letting the other person know how they make us feel'. But what perhaps is being spoken about by 'the relational' appears in the nooks and crannies that the particular theory can't reach, beyond conceptual totalising – and even beyond pluralism?

So, might we wonder what the relationship is between our distinguished contributors to this book and the methods they are putting forward; what qualities has it brought out in them which are helpful or unhelpful to their patients/ clients and indeed themselves and to what extent do these methods allow something magical to happen? Also, to speculate to probably the extreme, is it possible that these different psychotherapeutic methods have really come about in order to deal with different types of 'psychopathologies' in people who are psychological therapists? Enabling the therapist to be able to sit there for 50 minutes, minimising the damage their 'psychopathology' might do to the patient/client, whilst hopefully enabling something quite other to go to work and heal?

Perhaps a further advantage of having all these different approaches to the paranormal presented in this book is that you, as readers, may be able to modify your approach to the one that best suits your particular 'psychopathology'! Of course, here, as elsewhere, with so many different approaches provided in the psychological therapies, there is also the additional advantage of being able/disabled sometimes to project onto other approaches, aspects of ourselves which we have not worked through, and may not be able to be contained by our particular theorising!

As mentioned at the start of this chapter, the notion of relational therapy would appear to be of growing interest to counsellors, psychotherapists and psychoanalysts across all modalities. What though seems important is that there is something we might term 'paranormal' in 'the relational' which we can't fully name. As mentioned, certain teachers, as with psychological therapists, have it more and whilst training schools attempt to bring it out, we never really know what that 'it' is. For some it's relationality, for others it's inter-subjectivity or tacit, or transference/countertransference and so forth. None seem fully adequate to explain what it is we experience in the between. Whatever it is, it does though seem to fit Google's dictionary, as provided by Oxford Languages' definition of the paranormal as 'denoting events or phenomena...that are beyond the scope of normal scientific understanding'? I just prefer to call it 'the magic of the relational'.

In ending this chapter, I would like to reinforce its argument by returning to a quotation given in the introduction; but this time adding his next sentence with the all-important 'at least a part':

> 'A layman will no doubt find it hard to understand how pathological disorders of the body and mind can be eliminated by 'mere' words. He will feel that he is being asked to believe in magic. And he will not be so very wrong for the words which we use in our everyday speech are nothing more than watered down magic. But we shall have to follow a roundabout path in order to explain how science sets about restoring to words at least a part of their former magical power.' (Freud, 1890: 285)

Further in ending this book I will end with another quote from Freud (with again thanks to Brottman 2009 for bringing these to my attention) in support of notions of the paranormal including for example descriptions of hauntings (see for example Good & Rahimi, 2019) not being just metaphorical:

> "If I had to live my life over again, I should devote myself to psychical research, rather than psychoanalysis." Sigmund Freud, letter to Hereward Carrington, 1921 (cited in Brottman, 2009: 471)

Freud appears to have been more open to magic than most of his current successors, whilst simultaneously being wary of psychoanalysis not being tarnished by association. In doing so he enabled practices to evolve that both could claim scientific authority whilst allowing in enchanting mysteries. To conclude, I regard notions of the paranormal as being the essences of the psychological therapies. Various attempts have been made to move towards objectifying it from transference, countertransference to the relational to per-haps even phenomenology. But whatever, they appear currently, and likely forever, to be beyond the scope of normal scientific understanding. Hence, the 'magic of the relational' and perhaps with the help of Kierkegaard and the paranormal the most important question we might consider is: 'the person's, who is a psychotherapist, relation to the truth of psychotherapy or what it is to become a psychotherapist.'

References

Birtchnell, J. (1999). *Relating in psychotherapy: The application of a new theory*, Westport, CT: Praeger.

Beutler, L.E. and Harwood, T.M. (2002). What Is and Can Be Attributed to the Therapeutic Relationship? *Journal of Contemporary Psychotherapy*, 32, 25–33.

Brottman, M. (2009). Psychoanalysis and Magic: Then and Now. *American Imago*, 66(4), 471–489.

Freud, S. (1890) "Psychical (or Mental) Treatment". *The Standard Edition of the Complete Psychological Works of Sigmund Freud Volume XVII (1917–1919): An Infantile Neurosis and Other Works*, London: Hogarth Press, pp. 283–302.

Good, B. and Rahimi, S. (2019) Special Thematic Collection: Hauntology in Psychological Anthropology. *Ethos: The Journal of the Society for Psychological Anthropology*, 47(4), 407–529.

Greenberg, J. and Mitchell, S. (1983). *Object relations in psychoanalytic theory*, Cambridge, MA: Harvard University Press.

Hargaden, H. and Schwartz, J. (2007). Editorial. *European Journal of Psychotherapy & Counselling*, 9(1), 3–5.

Heidegger, M. (1962). *Being and time*. (J. Macquarrie and E. Robinson, Trans.). Oxford: Blackwell.

House, R. and Loewenthal, D. (Eds.). (2009). *Childhood, wellbeing and a therapeutic ethos*. London: Karnac.

James, W. (1890). *The principles of psychology* (Harvard Ed., Vol. 2), New York: Holt.

James, W. (1912). *Essays in radical empiricism* (R. Barton Perry Ed.), New York: Longmans, Green.

Kierkegaard, S. (1941) *Concluding unscientific postscript*, Princeton, NJ: Princeton University Press.

Loewenthal, D. (2007). *Case studies in relational research*, Basingstoke: Palgrave Macmillan.

Loewenthal, D. (2017) *Existential psychotherapy and counselling after postmodernism*, Abingdon: Routledge.

Loewenthal, D. and Samuels, A. (2014) *Relational psychotherapy, psychoanalysis and counselling: appraisals and reappraisals*, Abingdon: Routledge.

Luborsky, L. and Auerbach, A. (1985). "The therapeutic relationship in psychodynamic psychotherapy: The research evidence and its meaning for practice". In *Psychiatry update: The American Psychiatric Association annual review*. Edited by: R. Hales, and A. Frances, Vol. 4, pp. 550–561. Washington, DC: American Psychiatric Press.

Malan, D. (1999). *Individual psychotherapy and the science of psychodynamics*, 2nd, Oxford: Butterworth-Heinemann.

Merleau-Ponty, M. (1956). What Is Phenomenology? *Cross Currents*, 6, 59–70.

Mitchell, S. (1988). *Relational concepts in psychoanalysis: An integration*, Cambridge, MA: Harvard University Press.

Mitchell, S. and Aron, L. (1999). *Relational psychoanalysis: The emergence of a tradition*, Hillsdale, NJ: The Analytic Press.

Polanyi, M. (2009). *The Tacit Dimension Chicago*. Chicago: The University of Chicago Press.

Safran, J.D. and Muran, J.C. (2000). *Negotiating the therapeutic alliance: A relational treatment guide*, New York: Guilford Press.

Index

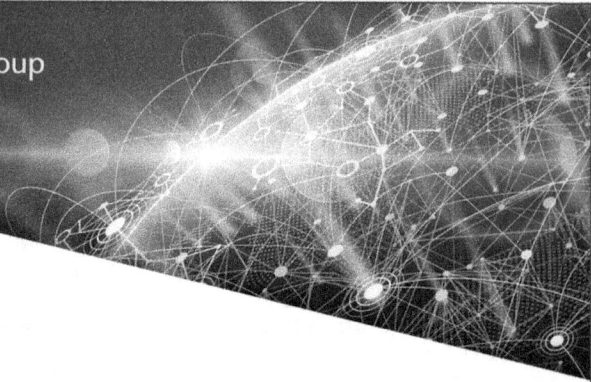

For Product Safety Concerns and Information please contact our EU
representative GPSR@taylorandfrancis.com
Taylor & Francis Verlag GmbH, Kaufingerstraße 24, 80331 München, Germany